Country Remedies
from pantry, field & garden

Karen Thesen

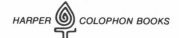
HARPER COLOPHON BOOKS

First edition HARPER & ROW, PUBLISHERS, INC 1979

ISBN   0 06 090687 1
LCCN   78 24701

Printed and bound in Great Britain at
William Clowes & Sons Limited, Beccles and London

Cover illustration by Ken Laidlaw
Line illustrations by Brigid Thesen

Contents

Dedicated to David and Ellinor

ACKNOWLEDGEMENTS

I would like to thank Philip and Jane Dunn and Hugh Van Dusen, without whose support and enthusiasm I would never have embarked on this project; Peter Gladwin and Jean Fisker of Expression Printers for their undying patience and help; Millicent Witherow whose enthusiasm has fired me from afar; and of course my sister Brigid for her marvellous illustrations, although at times I did have to resort to the old country remedy of tying her by the leg to the table to ensure the work was done . . .

Introduction

Having grown up in the wilds of the countryside with very few childhood ills and no medicine chest in the house, we learned early on just what to use to heal and soothe everyday cuts, grazes and bruises. Dock leaves grew in the fields and ditches in as great a profusion as the nettles whose sting they eased. Flowers, vegetables and herbs flourished in every available plot of earth. In the orchard, amongst the ancient fruit trees, were hives of bees who supplied plentiful honey for use all the year round.

We played hide and seek in the herbaceous borders, in and out of the tall plants of golden-rod, michaelmas daisies, lavender bushes and the twining periwinkle, all heavy with flowers and the buzzing of bees. Many of these plants were used by our mother and grandmother in the preparation of herbal teas and aromatic remedies for the treatment of minor ailments.

It is in that wild and free country upbringing that my interest in nature and natural things is firmly based. This led me to start collecting country remedies and cures, old wives' tales, superstitions, in fact anything that appealed to me either for its homely, natural content or merely for its curiosity value. Over the years I've referred to these scraps of information again and again and gradually built up quite an alchemist's cupboard.

I've found that the basic essentials are quite simply acquired: a pestle and mortar is most useful but not vital and in many cases the back of a wooden spoon on the side of a basin works almost as well; I have a pair of scales that measures in fractions of ounces up to only one pound; a set of measuring spoons and measuring cups; a length of butter muslin which is very reasonable to buy. I find that one yard lasts me for about a month or six weeks, depending on the season and how busy I am in the kitchen making lavender bags, aromatic bath bags, bran bags for toothache or earache, or whatever. You may need a fine sieve at times but on these occasions I use muslin again, to line an ordinary nylon sieve. A stock of screw-topped jars and plastic bottles is useful but you can make do with whatever you have to hand.

And then of course there are your ingredients, which you can build up gradually. Many things come from the kitchen shelves but you will need to buy some additional bits and pieces. I have found that the best thing is to get what you need for specific recipes and keep what is left in well-labelled, tightly-stoppered jars. You will soon discover your favourite herbs and those you want to keep always in stock. Many health food stores have a wide selection which you can buy loose and therefore much more cheaply than proprietary brands in fancy bottles. It is important to keep them all carefully labelled in sealed jars to prevent them going musty. For drying your own herbs see the herbal section. As for many of the oils and essences, I found that my local chemist (or drugstore) came up with all sorts of unexpected treasures at a very reasonable price, so you too might find it worth talking to your old-fashioned corner drugstore before you try the more expensive herbal stores.

During the background reading for this book I have learnt that in many cases scientific research now confirms many old wives' tales that had previously been dismissed as mere folklore. For example, in West Germany, research has recently shown that raw garlic can reduce the cholesterol level in the blood as well as kill bacteria that causes diseases such as diptheria and tuberculosis.

I have also learnt a lot about herbal history and legend. Before the rise of modern medicine curative plants were the mainstay of the physician's medicine chest. In the Middle Ages every monastery had its physick garden where monks tended the herbs and plants they used to cure the sick. Likewise countrywomen had their herb plots where they grew herbs for culinary and medicinal use. The American Indians had a great intuitive knowledge of many herbs, barks and roots and how to use them in the treatment of disease. Their native wisdom and medicinal skill were heavily relied on by the early pioneers of America. A century ago most housewives were acquainted with the remedial properties of herbs and taught their children to recognise the plants in the gardens and fields and learn their uses.

At the beginning of the last century travelling physicians were still seen in the English countryside, carrying their distilling equipment with them to prepare the wild herbs. They are still remembered today in the names of country pubs such as "The Green Man".

Many of the ancient herbalists believed that some plants had been stamped with the image of their properties to make it easier for the layman to recognise which plant to use for which malady; thus a herb with yellow sap was thought to be specifically to cure jaundice; one whose stem was rough and scaly would cure skin diseases; walnuts with their crenellations were good for the brain and weakness thereof; the liver-shaped leaves of the liverwort were a certain cure for liver diseases. Many of our familiar herbs got their popular names in this manner.

Flowers and plants have always been entangled with witchcraft and superstition. A witch would make her broomstick out of wood from the ash tree as that would protect her from drowning. She was thought to shelter in hawthorn hedges and emerge to pick her herbs in secrecy at certain phases of the moon and seasons of the year. All the poisonous plants are the witch's favourites and consequently the list of anti-witch plants is long. In Italy branches of juniper and in Germany, rowan, were hung over doorways to frighten witches away. Holy plants such as angelica and holly gave great protection especially when made up into the shape of a cross.

The history of herbalism can be traced right back to Theophrastus who wrote his *Enquiry into Plants* in about 320 BC. Pliny's *Natural History* written some 300 years later, lists and classifies plants of every kind. Dioscorides in *De Materia Medica* mentions some 500 healing herbs and his theories have been frequently referred to by succeeding herbalists. Enthusiasm and interest in curative plants then lapsed until the sixteenth century when a number of new works were published. William Turner published *A New Herball* in 1551 and was followed by John Gerard (1597) whose *Herball* has become one of the standard works, along with that of Nicholas Culpeper whose *Complete Herbal and English Physician Enlarged* was published in 1649. These are all well-known works that are constantly referred to in modern herbalism, but the best of the modern herbals is Mrs M Grieve's *A Modern Herbal* (1931) which has now become the authority and is endlessly fascinating and interesting to read and full of worthwhile information should you wish to pursue the subject. Also, the marvellous specialist publisher, The C W Daniel Company Ltd of London, publishes countless interesting and useful books on all aspects of nature cure, herbalism, homoeopathy.

This collection of remedies and cures offer an interesting and successful way of treating a variety of common ailments. The remedies are simple, use familiar ingredients and can be fun to prepare and take. Of course I am not advocating self-diagnosis and treatment in the event of any more serious illness, but I am suggesting that the use of these country remedies in preference to reaching for the aspirins, indigestion tablets or cough syrups for the treatment of minor complaints, may well cure you in a natural, easy way without any side effects.

This is a book that is meant to be enjoyed and made use of. I have divided it into five sections, mainly for interest and ease of reference, but in many cases the decision has been rather arbitrary as to which section a certain remedy fits into. The sections themselves overlap each other and many remedies would be equally happy under more than one heading. I have therefore added a good, clear index with plenty of cross references for all the remedies and ailments mentioned in the book. It has been great fun and very satisfying compiling this book and trying everything out and I am delighted to offer this selection of reliable, enjoyable and surprisingly effective country remedies to a wider public.

K.T.

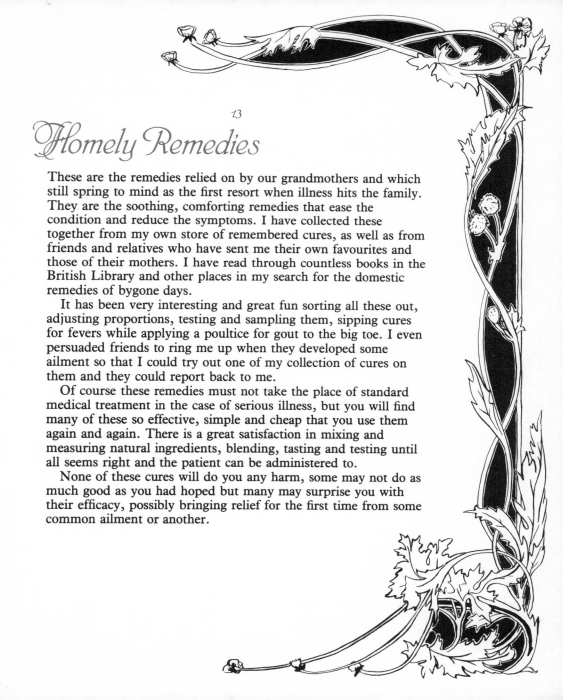

Homely Remedies

These are the remedies relied on by our grandmothers and which still spring to mind as the first resort when illness hits the family. They are the soothing, comforting remedies that ease the condition and reduce the symptoms. I have collected these together from my own store of remembered cures, as well as from friends and relatives who have sent me their own favourites and those of their mothers. I have read through countless books in the British Library and other places in my search for the domestic remedies of bygone days.

It has been very interesting and great fun sorting all these out, adjusting proportions, testing and sampling them, sipping cures for fevers while applying a poultice for gout to the big toe. I even persuaded friends to ring me up when they developed some ailment so that I could try out one of my collection of cures on them and they could report back to me.

Of course these remedies must not take the place of standard medical treatment in the case of serious illness, but you will find many of these so effective, simple and cheap that you use them again and again. There is a great satisfaction in mixing and measuring natural ingredients, blending, tasting and testing until all seems right and the patient can be administered to.

None of these cures will do you any harm, some may not do as much good as you had hoped but many may surprise you with their efficacy, possibly bringing relief for the first time from some common ailment or another.

Mrs Beeton's Cold Cure

Mrs Beeton in her *Book of Household Management* (1861) has sections which cover every eventuality in the home. Some of her ideas and suggestions in *The Doctor* section sound rather alarming to the modern reader and she did seem over-fond of leeches. But this cure of hers is surprisingly pleasant in spite of the pungent smell of linseed oil, which virtually disappears during preparation, and contains all the traditional ingredients for warding off colds. Mrs Beeton assures us "The worst cold is generally cured by this remedy in two or three days, and, if taken in time, it is considered infallible."

3 tablespoons linseed oil
1 ounce (3 tablespoons) raisins
8-inch piece of liquorice root
1 pint (2½ cups) water
1 ounce (2 tablespoons) sugar
1 teaspoon rum
1 teaspoon lemon juice

Put the linseed oil, raisins and liquorice root into the water and simmer gently over a low heat until reduced by half. Stir in the sugar. Cool, strain and add the rum and lemon juice. Sip a teaspoonful, tepid, as required or whenever the cough is troublesome.

A Fever Mixture

This mixture is recommended in all cases of fever induced by mild burns, sunburn, painful sprains.

1½ teaspoons cream of tartar
½ teaspoon lemon juice
1 pint (2½ cups) warm water

Combine all the ingredients and give the patient a wineglassful as necessary. You may prefer this with the addition of ½ teaspoon honey.

Eucalyptus Inhalant for catarrh in the head

The leathery pendulous leaves of this fast-growing tree are studded with glands that produce the fragrant volatile oil so well known all over the world.

½ cup boiling water
a few drops oil of eucalyptus

Pour the boiling water into a basin and stir in the oil of eucalyptus. Lean over the basin and cover your head and the basin with a large towel, thereby enclosing the fumes. Inhale the steam for 10 minutes, keeping the eyes tightly closed.

Garlic Syrup for asthma

Many marvellous effects and healing powers have been attributed to garlic. This syrup is invaluable for asthma, hoarseness, coughs, difficulty of breathing and most disorders of the lungs.

3 whole heads of garlic
1 pint (2½ cups) water
½ pint (1¼ cups) cider vinegar
2 ounces (¼ cup) sugar

Break the heads of garlic into separate cloves and peel these. Place in a saucepan with the water and simmer gently until reduced by half. Remove the garlic, add the vinegar and sugar to the water and continue boiling until reduced to a syrup. Meanwhile put the garlic cloves into a jar and pour the syrup over. The dose is 1 or 2 cloves of garlic to be taken with a spoonful of the syrup every morning.

Watercress Asthma Remedy

A popular prescription for spasmodic asthma, according to a correspondent in the *Medical Times* (1868) is to eat heartily of watercress.

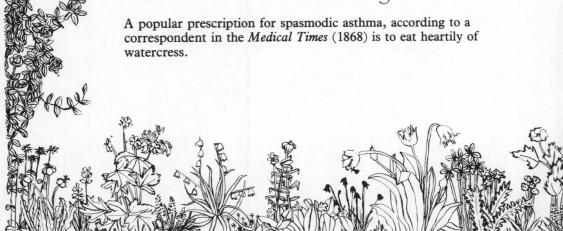

Onion Cough Syrup

6 medium-sized onions, peeled & finely chopped
½ cup honey

Put the onions and honey into the top of a double boiler, or into a basin over a pan of boiling water. Cover and simmer gently for 2 hours. Strain and take the oniony honey frequently, preferably warm.

Chestnut Leaf Infusion
for coughs

The leaves of the sweet chestnut tree must be picked in June or July when they are in peak condition, and then carefully dried.
This infusion is particularly useful in cases of convulsive coughs, such as whooping cough, and in other irritable conditions of the respiratory organs.

1 pint (2½ cups) boiling water
1 ounce (½ cup) dried sweet chestnut leaves

Pour the boiling water over the dried leaves and allow to stand for 20 minutes. Strain and administer 1 tablespoonful 3 or 4 times a day.

Sunflower Syrup
for chest infections

This is as delicious as it sounds. Sunflower seeds have diuretic and expectorant qualities and when crushed are rich in an excellent, light oil. This oil can be used in cases of bronchial infections, colds and coughs, being given in doses of 10 to 15 drops, 2 or 3 times a day. Or, this special mixture, which is much more palatable, can be given.

2 ounces (½ cup) sunflower seeds
2 pints (5 cups) water
2 ounces (¼ cup) sugar
7 tablespoons (¾ cup) gin

Boil the sunflower seeds in the water until reduced to ¾ pint (2 cups). Strain, stir in the sugar, then add the gin. This delightful preparation should be given 3 or 4 times a day in doses of 1 to 2 teaspoonfuls. You will find that the difficulty here is in restricting yourself to the prescribed dosage.

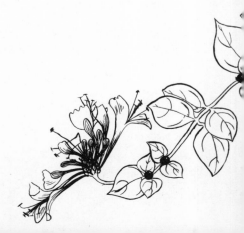

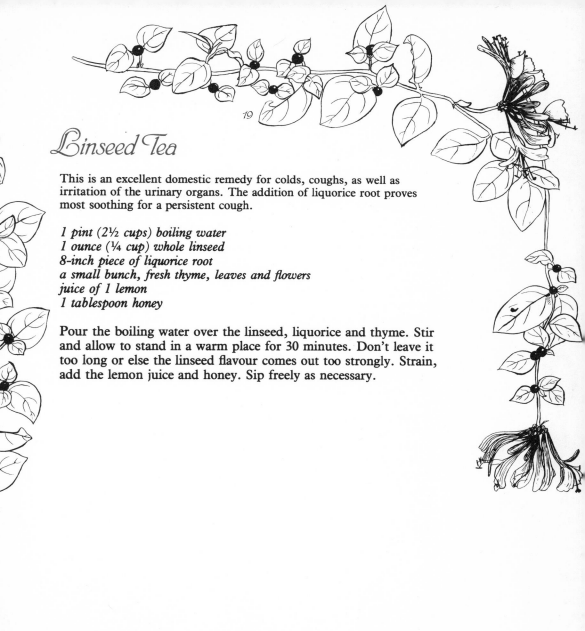

Linseed Tea

This is an excellent domestic remedy for colds, coughs, as well as irritation of the urinary organs. The addition of liquorice root proves most soothing for a persistent cough.

1 pint (2½ cups) boiling water
1 ounce (¼ cup) whole linseed
8-inch piece of liquorice root
a small bunch, fresh thyme, leaves and flowers
juice of 1 lemon
1 tablespoon honey

Pour the boiling water over the linseed, liquorice and thyme. Stir and allow to stand in a warm place for 30 minutes. Don't leave it too long or else the linseed flavour comes out too strongly. Strain, add the lemon juice and honey. Sip freely as necessary.

A Norfolk Cold Cure

Again, garlic's curative powers are called upon for a traditional remedy. The penetrating odour of the garlic is said to be so diffusive that even when applied to the soles of the feet, its odour is carried on the breath.

6 cloves garlic, peeled
4 ounces (½ cup) white lard (shortening)

Crush the garlic and mash it into the lard. Spread the mixture over the soles of the patient's feet which should be kept warm by covering with a thick warmed towel. It is advisable to rest the feet on a thick pile of newspapers to absorb any grease. Repeat as often as necessary until cured.

Hot Lemon & Honey

A tasty, health-giving alternative to numerous cups of tea and coffee during the day is hot lemon and honey. Coffee gives me headaches and tea stains my teeth so it is with great delight I turn to this refreshing drink which is made by adding a teaspoon of lemon juice or a slice of lemon to a glass of hot water and sweetening with a teaspoon of honey.
It is also excellent in all cases of nausea and, with the addition of 3 whole cloves or a ½-inch piece of stick cinnamon, is a good remedy for coughs, colds and sore throats.

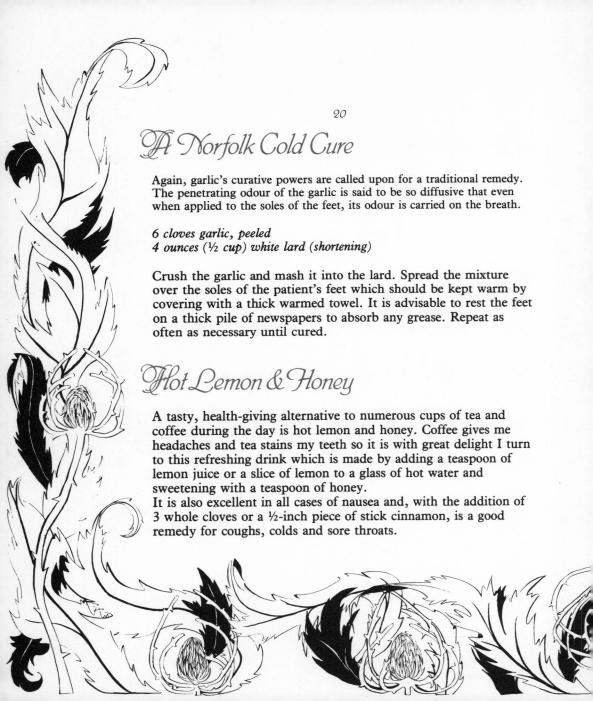

Hot Potato Water
for rheumatism

There was a firm conviction years ago that a sure way to avoid rheumatism was to carry a raw potato in your pocket at all times. Recently, this has been shown to be based on more than mere superstition – raw potato juice has been used successfully in the treatment of rheumatism and gout. This hot potato water has been a popular remedy for years.

1 pound (2 cups) potatoes, diced
2 pints (5 cups) water

Put the diced potatoes, which should be left unpeeled, into a saucepan with the water and bring slowly to the boil. Continue boiling gently until the water has reduced by half. Steep clean cloths or bandages in the water, wring out and apply, as hot as possible, to the affected parts.

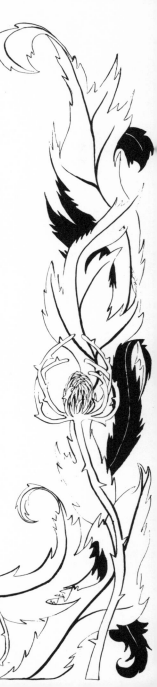

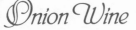

Onion Wine

This is an excellent remedy for many ailments, particularly anaemia, water retention and general debility. It is a fine tonic and you can take it freely as a preventative measure – 1 tablespoon every morning during the winter months.

4½ tablespoons clear honey
1 pint (2½ cups) white wine
2 onions, finely chopped

Stir the honey into the wine until dissolved, then add the onions. Cover and leave in a cool, dark place for 48 hours, stirring frequently. Strain and bottle. The dose is 1 tablespoon to be taken 3 or 4 times a day.

Barley Water

There was always a jug of barley water in the fridge when I was a child; with the addition of lemon and honey it was a favourite and refreshing drink. As the traditional beverage for invalids and children it is also good for feverish conditions and in infections of the respiratory organs and general 'chestiness'.
Barley water can be used to dilute cows' milk for young infants as it prevents the formation of hard lumps of curd in the stomach.

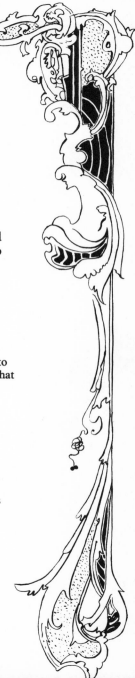

1 tablespoon pearl barley
1¼ pints (3 cups) water

Wash the barley in a sieve under running water, then soak
overnight in the water. Bring to the boil and simmer gently,
stirring constantly until the barley is soft and the liquid reduced
by one third. Strain. Salt, lemon juice or honey can be added to
taste.

Rice Water

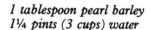

This has long been the country remedy for diarrhoea because of its
soothing action on the intestines. And should you be unlucky enough to
contract hepatitis (inflammation of the liver), rice water should be all that
you take for the first few days.

2 tablespoons brown rice
2 pints (5 cups) water
1 tablespoon honey

Bring the rice to the boil in the water and boil for 30 minutes.
Strain through a sieve and sweeten to taste with honey. Some
people like to add about 1 tablespoon of lemon juice to give this
bland drink a bit more bite. This water can be taken freely, as
desired, a small glassful at a time.

Albumen Water

A traditional remedy for an upset stomach and particularly mild for
children (but give without the brandy).

1 egg white
1 cup water
sugar to taste
½ teaspoon brandy (optional)

Add the egg white to the water and stir slowly with a spoon for 5
minutes. Don't use a fork and don't stir too fast or else you will
break the albumen up. Strain through a sieve, sweeten to taste
and add the brandy if desired. If has a very light flavour and is a
most welcome drink when you feel nauseous or bilious.
Alternatively, use the unsweetened, unflavoured albumen water to
dilute rose-hip or redcurrant syrup.

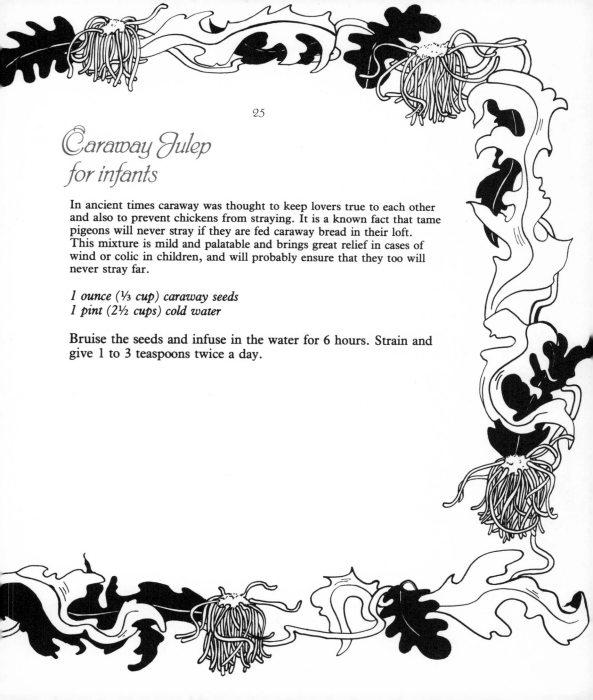

Caraway Julep
for infants

In ancient times caraway was thought to keep lovers true to each other and also to prevent chickens from straying. It is a known fact that tame pigeons will never stray if they are fed caraway bread in their loft. This mixture is mild and palatable and brings great relief in cases of wind or colic in children, and will probably ensure that they too will never stray far.

1 ounce (⅓ cup) caraway seeds
1 pint (2½ cups) cold water

Bruise the seeds and infuse in the water for 6 hours. Strain and give 1 to 3 teaspoons twice a day.

Oat Gruel

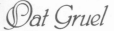

This is a fine drink to restore those convalescing from a debilitating illness. It is soothing and restorative as well as having mild diuretic properties.
You can use everyday porridge oats to make this but the less refined the oats the better.

7 ounces (2 cups) oats
3 pints (7½ cups) water
2 tablespoons honey

Wash the oats thoroughly in plenty of cold water then put them in a saucepan with the water and bring to the boil. Simmer until reduced by one third, strain through a fine sieve and stir in the honey. This soothing, warming drink with its slightly gluey consistency can be taken freely. It is much more palatable warm than cold when it takes on an even thicker gluey consistency reminiscent of cold porridge.
Alternative flavourings can be lemon juice, a little white wine or a few raisins which should be added right at the beginning of the brewing.

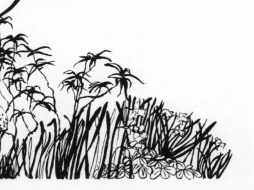

Bran Tea

Bran is rich in minerals and iron and this tea is an excellent way of obtaining extra iron naturally if you suffer from anaemia. Certainly, my elder sister religiously drank a cup of this tea daily during her pregnancy and remained blooming throughout.

2 tablespoons wheat bran
1 pint (2½ cups) boiling water
1 tablespoon honey
1 tablespoon lemon juice

Add the bran to the water in a saucepan and bring to the boil. Simmer for 15 minutes, then strain through a sieve and stir in the honey and lemon juice. Take as desired.

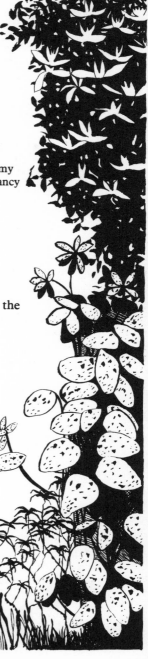

Vinegar Gargle for sore throat

1 teaspoon salt
½ cup vinegar
1 cup warm water

Dissolve the salt in the vinegar, add the water and use this mixture to gargle every 15 minutes until cured. Be careful not to swallow it as it will make you retch.

Cereal Broth

A good source of nourishment in cases of infantile gastro-enteritis and also for those convalescing after a serious illness.

½ cup wheat
½ cup oats
½ cup barley
1¼ pints (3 cups) water
honey to taste

Grind the grains together in a food mill or pestle and mortar. Take 4 tablespoons of this mixture, add to the water and bring to the boil. Continue boiling until reduced by one third, strain and sweeten to taste with honey.

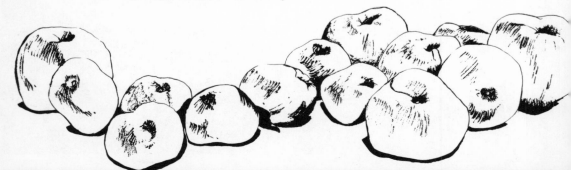

Apple Water

An excellent recipe for a suitable drink to be taken in all cases of feverishness. It is important to use a good, light honey so that it doesn't flavour this delicate refreshing water too strongly.

3 cooking apples
1½ pints (3¾ cups) water
2 tablespoons honey

Core and slice the apples without peeling and place in a saucepan with the water. Bring to the boil and simmer until the apples are just beginning to break down. Remove from the heat, strain without pressing the apple purée through the sieve, and stir the honey into the liquid.
You can take this apple water, cold, as often as required.

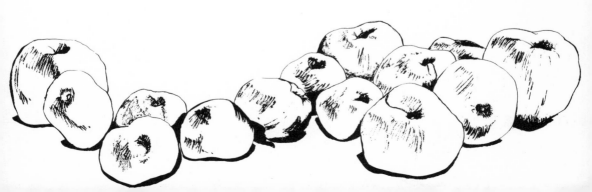

Arrowroot Gruel

The fine white powder known as arrowroot is the starch extracted from the rhizomes of a herbaceous perennial that grows widely in the West Indies and Central America. The local people applied the mashed rhizomes to wounds from poisoned arrows, hence the name.
The blandness and digestibility of arrowroot makes it valuable in cases of bowel complaints or stomach upsets and to nourish convalescents.

1 tablespoon arrowroot
1 pint (2½ cups) milk
1 tablespoon sugar or honey
a few drops vanilla (optional)

Mix the arrowroot to a smooth paste with a little of the milk. Bring the rest of the milk to the boil and blend into the arrowroot paste. Return to the heat and stir continuously until the milk has thickened slightly and just begins to boil again. Remove from the heat and stir in the sugar or honey and vanilla to flavour if used. This can be taken whenever desired.

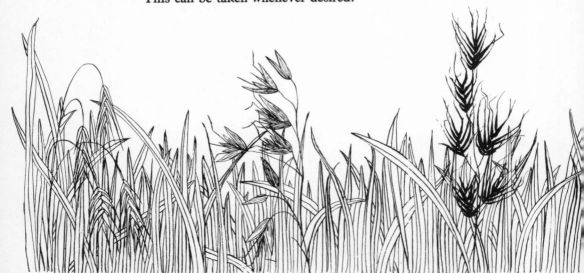

Slippery Elm Food

Only the inner bark of this small American tree is used medicinally. Made into a thin gruel it is a wholesome and sustaining food for invalids and infants. It can also be taken in cases of irritation of the mucous membranes of the stomach or intestines as it is bland, soothing and nutritious.

1 teaspoon slippery elm powder
1 pint (2½ cups) boiling water

Mix the slippery elm powder into a thin paste with a little cold water. Then pour on the boiling water, stirring constantly. I find the mixture nearly always goes lumpy, so I resort to giving it a quick whizz in the electric blender. If desired, add a pinch of ground cinnamon, grated nutmeg or lemon rind. Take unsweetened 3 times a day for gastritis, mucous colitis and enteritis. Taken at night it will induce sleep.

My favourite way of making it is to beat 1 egg into 1 teaspoon of the powder, then pour on 1 pint (2½ cups) boiling milk, whisking constantly. This can then be sweetened with brown sugar or honey and is a much more body-building and tasty way of having the drink.

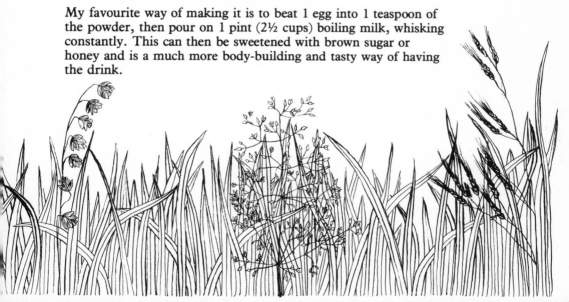

Elderflower Vinegar

This is an old recipe for a delicious variation to wine vinegar. Weakly diluted with water it makes a refreshing drink when you have a high temperature, and in a stronger solution is an excellent gargle for a sore throat.

elderflowers, fresh or dried
1 pint (2½ cups) cider vinegar

Pick the flowers over and remove the stalks and dead heads. Pack as many as possible into an earthenware jar and pour the vinegar over. Seal the jar and store in a warm place for 8 days. Shake the jar occasionally during this time. Strain through a sieve lined with muslin and keep in a well-stoppered bottle.

Lavender Vinegar

This makes a refreshing toilet water which if applied to the temples can bring you great relief from headaches caused by fatigue and exhaustion.

8 ounces (1¾ cups) dried lavender flowers
1 pint (1¼ cups) cider vinegar
½ pint (1¼ cups) rosewater

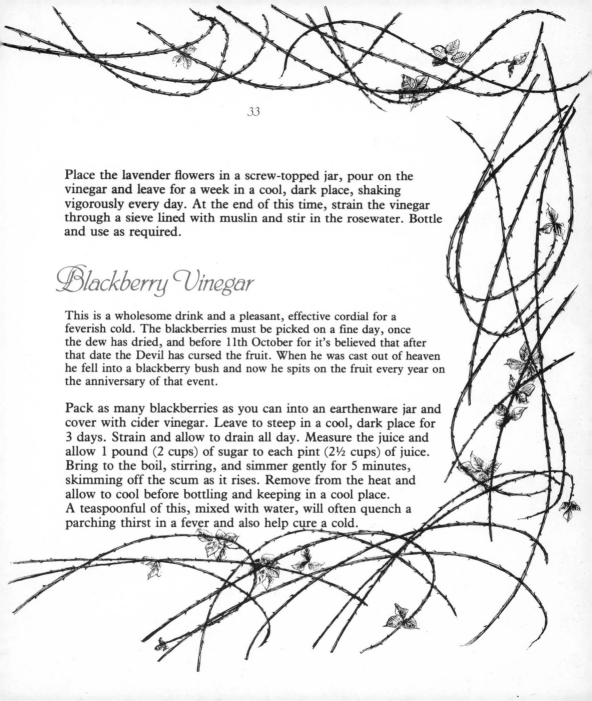

Place the lavender flowers in a screw-topped jar, pour on the vinegar and leave for a week in a cool, dark place, shaking vigorously every day. At the end of this time, strain the vinegar through a sieve lined with muslin and stir in the rosewater. Bottle and use as required.

Blackberry Vinegar

This is a wholesome drink and a pleasant, effective cordial for a feverish cold. The blackberries must be picked on a fine day, once the dew has dried, and before 11th October for it's believed that after that date the Devil has cursed the fruit. When he was cast out of heaven he fell into a blackberry bush and now he spits on the fruit every year on the anniversary of that event.

Pack as many blackberries as you can into an earthenware jar and cover with cider vinegar. Leave to steep in a cool, dark place for 3 days. Strain and allow to drain all day. Measure the juice and allow 1 pound (2 cups) of sugar to each pint (2½ cups) of juice. Bring to the boil, stirring, and simmer gently for 5 minutes, skimming off the scum as it rises. Remove from the heat and allow to cool before bottling and keeping in a cool place. A teaspoonful of this, mixed with water, will often quench a parching thirst in a fever and also help cure a cold.

Raspberry Vinegar

This makes a useful gargle for sore throats and also, when diluted with water, is an excellent cooling drink in summer. It can also be taken when you have a fever or raised temperature.

10 ounces (2 cups) raspberries
1 pint (2½ cups) white wine vinegar
8 ounces (1 cup) sugar

Place the raspberries in a bowl and pour over the vinegar. Stir and cover and leave in a cool place for 3 to 4 days. After this time place in a saucepan, add the sugar and bring gently to the boil, stirring. Simmer for 15-20 minutes, remove from the heat and allow to cool. Strain, pressing as much juice as possible through the sieve. Bottle and use as required.

Leek Ointment

This is recommended as one of the best applications for severe sprains and aches. It can also be used to help heal burns and scalds – but be sure not to apply it directly after a burn as oil or grease of any sort delays the cooling of the skin and can intensify the burn.

3 leeks, cleaned & chopped
3 tablespoons coconut butter

Simmer the leeks in boiling water until quite soft and tender. Drain off the liquid and press the leeks through a sieve. Stir the coconut butter into the leek purée and allow to cool. The resulting light green ointment with its slight oniony smell can be applied liberally.

Green Elder Ointment

Granny must have known about elder leaves for she used to crush them and wrap them around our summer bruises.
This delicately-coloured ointment works wonders for bruises, sprains, chillblains and even for wounds where the skin is broken.

8 ounces (3 cups) fresh elder leaves
8 ounces (1 cup) lard (shortening)
2½ ounces (½ cup) shredded suet

Put all the ingredients together into a saucepan and heat gently until liquified and the green colour is extracted from the leaves. Strain through a sieve lined with muslin and weighted with a saucer slightly smaller in diameter than the sieve, so as to press through as much of the mixture as possible. Bottle while still warm and allow to cool before placing the tops on the bottles. Store in a cool place and use as necessary.

Elderflower Ointment

Cheaper and more effective than many cosmetic after-sun preparations, this mild and cooling ointment is of great relief when used on skin that has been over-exposed to the sun.

2 handfuls fresh elderflowers
4 ounces (½ cup) lard (shortening)

Strip the flowers from the stalks and heat gently with the lard (shortening), stirring constantly. Simmer for 15 minutes, then strain while still warm through a sieve into jars or bottles.

A Head Rub

Massaging the scalp increases local circulation and is very beneficial to both hair and scalp. Rosemary is exceptional for hair care, being a natural conditioner adding lustre to the hair and preventing dandruff and hair loss. This aromatic oil rub is a pleasure to use and well worth the extra few minutes before shampooing.

2 tablespoons almond oil
2 teaspoons oil of rosemary

Put the almond oil into a cup and stand the cup in a pan of boiling water. Heat the oil and add the oil of rosemary. Take care not to get the oil too hot as the scalp can be very sensitive. Massage the warm oil well into the scalp before washing the hair, preferably with a rosemary shampoo.

An Ancient Method
to preserve hair & make it grow thick

1 cup rosemary flowers & tops
2 pints (5 cups) white wine
8 ounces (⅔ cup) honey
¼ pint (⅔ cup) sweet almond oil

Steep the rosemary in the wine for 8 hours or overnight. Add the honey and stir until dissolved, add the sweet almond oil and stir the mixture thoroughly. Put about 2-3 tablespoons of this mixture into a cup, stand it in a pan of water over the heat and warm it to blood temperature. Massage the scalp with this and comb it through the hair. Leave on for at least 30 minutes before washing off.

To Cure Baldness

For this you need beef-bone marrow and the best bones to get to extract the marrow are the large, long, thigh bones. Ask your butcher to cut them into pieces about 6 inches long and then it is an easy task to scoop the crumbly marrow out with a teaspoon or skewer.

1 ounce (½ cup) dried elderflowers
1 pint (2½ cups) boiling water
beef-bone marrow

Put the elderflowers into a saucepan, pour on the boiling water and simmer gently for 1 hour. Strain off the flowers, and continue simmering the liquid until reduced to a thick syrup. Add an equal amount of beef-bone marrow, stirring well. Remove from the heat and continue stirring until cool and stiff. Rub well into the scalp night and morning and you certainly deserve a glossy, shining head of hair.

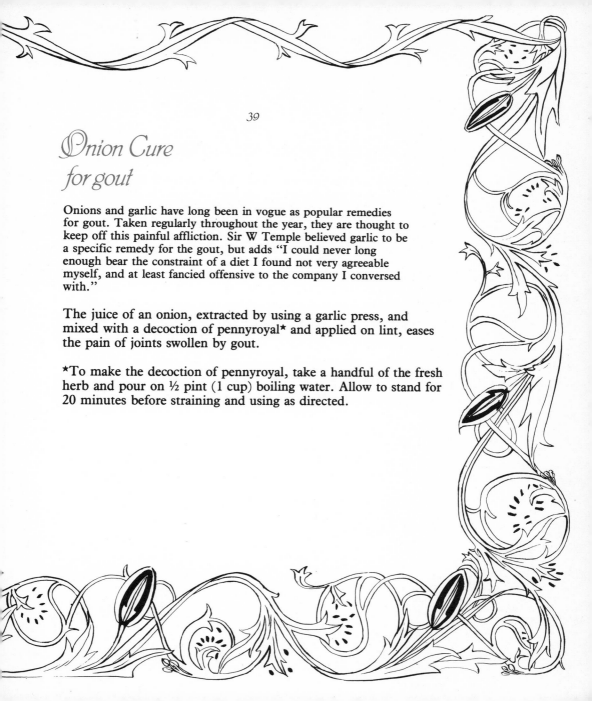

Onion Cure
for gout

Onions and garlic have long been in vogue as popular remedies
for gout. Taken regularly throughout the year, they are thought to
keep off this painful affliction. Sir W Temple believed garlic to be
a specific remedy for the gout, but adds "I could never long
enough bear the constraint of a diet I found not very agreeable
myself, and at least fancied offensive to the company I conversed
with."

The juice of an onion, extracted by using a garlic press, and
mixed with a decoction of pennyroyal* and applied on lint, eases
the pain of joints swollen by gout.

*To make the decoction of pennyroyal, take a handful of the fresh
herb and pour on ½ pint (1 cup) boiling water. Allow to stand for
20 minutes before straining and using as directed.

Slippery Elm Poultice for rheumatic joints

The Red Indians have long used powdered slippery elm as a healing salve because it is soothing and reduces pain and inflammation. Here, the slippery elm is mixed with bran which helps retain the heat.

½ pint (1¼ cups) vinegar
4 ounces (1 cup) slippery elm powder
1½ ounces (1 cup) bran

Heat the vinegar in a saucepan, stir in the slippery elm powder and bran and mix into a paste. Spread on to a linen cloth, fold over and apply, as hot as can be borne, to the painful joint.

Honey & Nettle Poultice for rheumatic joints

Nettles have since ancient times been used as a remedy for rheumatism – the afflicted joints would be rubbed or beaten with fresh nettles for a few minutes each day and the condition would improve. However, this honey and nettle poultice is a less painful way of obtaining the same results.

1 large (gloved) handful nettle tops
1 pint (2½ cups) water
2 tablespoons honey

Chop the nettle tops, put into a saucepan with the water and bring to the boil. Simmer for 10 minutes. Strain. Soak a pad of lint in this hot liquid, squeeze out the excess liquid. Warm the honey and spread on to the lint. Wrap the painful joint with this poultice and bind loosely with a dry bandage.

Honey Poultice for boils

Honey is a natural healer, having bacterial power which can draw out and overcome the infection.

1 tablespoon honey
1 tablespoon cod-liver oil

Mix the honey and cod-liver oil together. Spread on a clean piece of linen. Apply to the boil and bind with clean cloth or bandages. Renew the dressing every 8 hours.

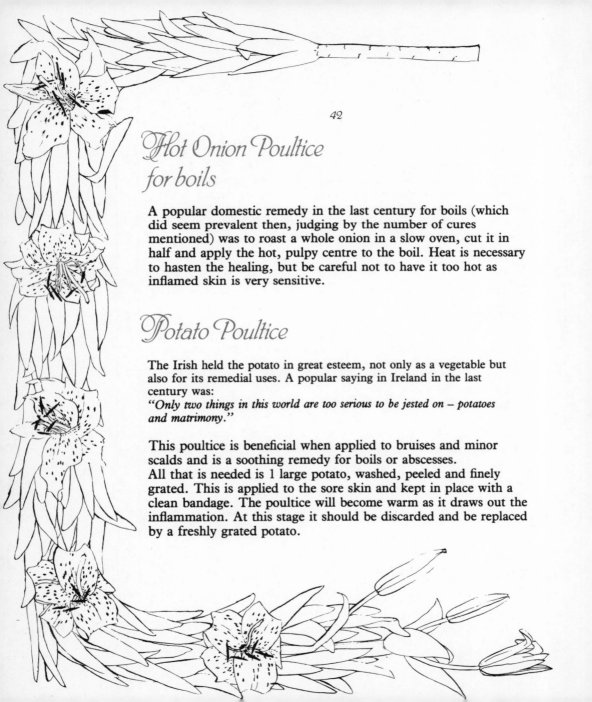

Hot Onion Poultice for boils

A popular domestic remedy in the last century for boils (which did seem prevalent then, judging by the number of cures mentioned) was to roast a whole onion in a slow oven, cut it in half and apply the hot, pulpy centre to the boil. Heat is necessary to hasten the healing, but be careful not to have it too hot as inflamed skin is very sensitive.

Potato Poultice

The Irish held the potato in great esteem, not only as a vegetable but also for its remedial uses. A popular saying in Ireland in the last century was:
"Only two things in this world are too serious to be jested on – potatoes and matrimony."

This poultice is beneficial when applied to bruises and minor scalds and is a soothing remedy for boils or abscesses.
All that is needed is 1 large potato, washed, peeled and finely grated. This is applied to the sore skin and kept in place with a clean bandage. The poultice will become warm as it draws out the inflammation. At this stage it should be discarded and be replaced by a freshly grated potato.

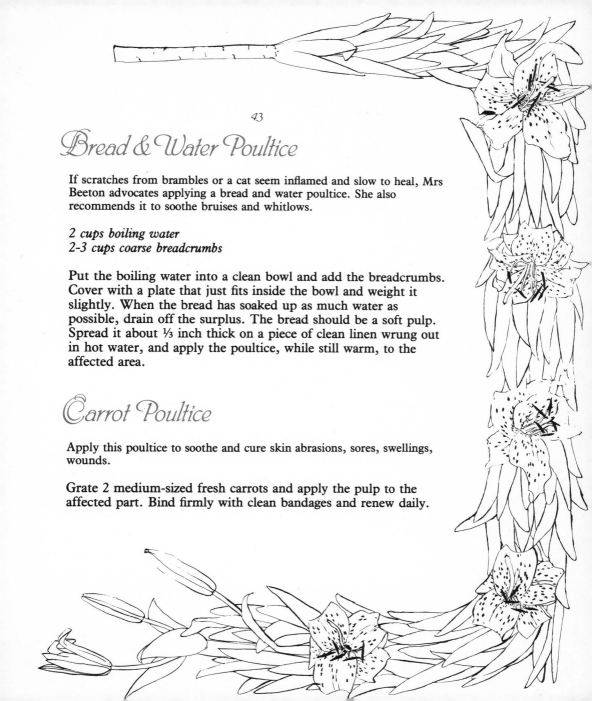

Bread & Water Poultice

If scratches from brambles or a cat seem inflamed and slow to heal, Mrs Beeton advocates applying a bread and water poultice. She also recommends it to soothe bruises and whitlows.

2 cups boiling water
2-3 cups coarse breadcrumbs

Put the boiling water into a clean bowl and add the breadcrumbs. Cover with a plate that just fits inside the bowl and weight it slightly. When the bread has soaked up as much water as possible, drain off the surplus. The bread should be a soft pulp. Spread it about ⅓ inch thick on a piece of clean linen wrung out in hot water, and apply the poultice, while still warm, to the affected area.

Carrot Poultice

Apply this poultice to soothe and cure skin abrasions, sores, swellings, wounds.

Grate 2 medium-sized fresh carrots and apply the pulp to the affected part. Bind firmly with clean bandages and renew daily.

Cornflour (Cornstarch) Poultice

Rather surprisingly cornflour (cornstarch) has healing properties and when made into a poultice is very soothing and healing for surface abrasions and bruises.

2 tablespoons cornflour (cornstarch)
3 teaspoons castor oil

Add the castor oil to the cornflour (cornstarch) and mix into a thick paste. Spread this paste on to a damp, clean cotton cloth about the size of a man's handkerchief. Fold over and apply to the affected part.

Fig & Potato Poultice

This is an excellent poultice to reduce swelling and ease painful joints.

4 ounces (⅔ cup) dried figs, chopped
1 medium-sized potato, grated
2 teaspoons glycerine

Combine the chopped figs, grated potato and glycerine and mix to form a paste. Spread this on to a clean damp cloth, fold over and apply as necessary.

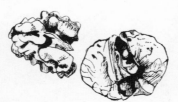
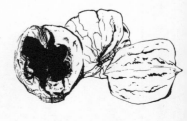

An Aromatic Bag
for toothache or earache

This warm bag applied externally to a sore ear or tooth does bring great relief and smells good at the same time.

1 stick of cinnamon
½ nutmeg, grated
2 blades of mace
4 cloves

Pound all the ingredients together in a pestle and mortar until coarsely powdered. Sew up in a small muslin bag, heat in a low oven and apply to the painful part.
I find this particularly useful for earache in children. I put a few drops of slightly warmed almond oil into the ear, plug it with cotton wool and then give the child this warm aromatic bag to hold pressed to the ear. They do find it very soothing.

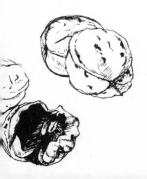
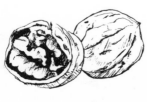
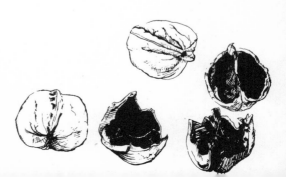

Caraway Poultice
for earache

Caraway was believed to prevent the theft of anything that contained it so it was used extensively in baking in ancient times and was also put into precious vessels and utensils around the house to keep them safe.

1 ounce (⅓ cup) caraway seeds
2 ounces (1 cup) soft, fresh breadcrumbs

Pound the caraway seeds in a pestle and mortar. Add the breadcrumbs, which should be from a hot, newly-baked loaf. If hot crumbs aren't used, heat the poultice slightly in the oven before wrapping in a piece of muslin and applying to the painful ear.

Bran Bag for earache

1 handful bran
1 handful coarse salt

Mix the bran and salt together and tie up in a muslin bag. Heat gently in a low oven and once warmed through, but not too hot, apply to the sore ear.

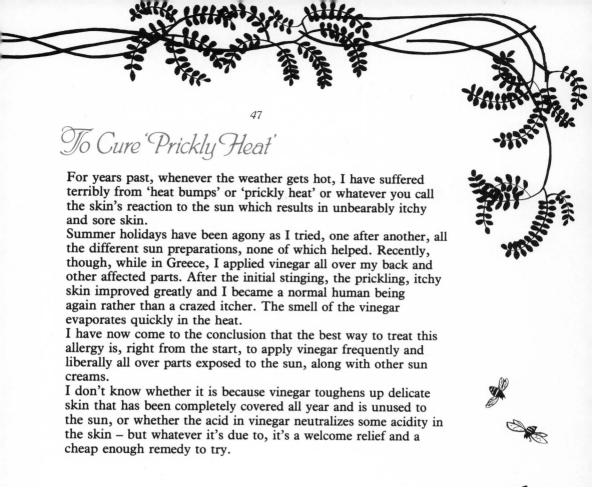

To Cure 'Prickly Heat'

For years past, whenever the weather gets hot, I have suffered terribly from 'heat bumps' or 'prickly heat' or whatever you call the skin's reaction to the sun which results in unbearably itchy and sore skin.

Summer holidays have been agony as I tried, one after another, all the different sun preparations, none of which helped. Recently, though, while in Greece, I applied vinegar all over my back and other affected parts. After the initial stinging, the prickling, itchy skin improved greatly and I became a normal human being again rather than a crazed itcher. The smell of the vinegar evaporates quickly in the heat.

I have now come to the conclusion that the best way to treat this allergy is, right from the start, to apply vinegar frequently and liberally all over parts exposed to the sun, along with other sun creams.

I don't know whether it is because vinegar toughens up delicate skin that has been completely covered all year and is unused to the sun, or whether the acid in vinegar neutralizes some acidity in the skin – but whatever it's due to, it's a welcome relief and a cheap enough remedy to try.

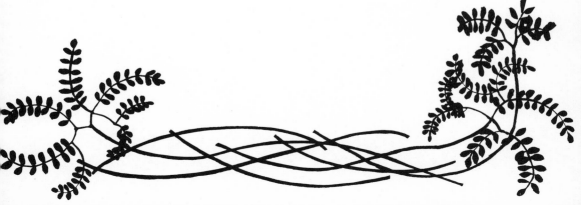

Apple Honey

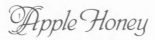

This is a delicious preserve and an excellent way of taking the goodness of apples, the chief dietetic value of which is the malic and tartaric acids in them. These acids are of especial benefit to sedentary people, who are liable to liver disorders, and they also neutralize the acid products of gout and indigestion.

To make the apple honey you simply take a quantity of eating apples (windfalls are ideal) peel, core and slice them and simmer gently with a little water but no sugar over a very low heat for 3 hours or more until thick, brown and very sweet.

A Toothache Remedy

An ancient cure for toothache was to burn brandy on a pewter plate and breathe in the fumes. Certainly worth trying but it seems a pity to waste the brandy – I would rather drink it to numb the pain . . . Oil of cloves has long been renowned for its beneficial effect on an aching tooth. A wad of cotton wool soaked in oil of cloves and held on the aching tooth brings great relief – or you can try my favourite toothache remedy.

1 tablespoon clear honey
5 whole cloves

Heat the honey in a saucepan and add the cloves. Stir and remove the cloves and chew them slowly and gently, rolling them around the aching tooth. The chewing releases the essential oil, which is the magic ingredient.

Sweet Almond Emulsion for disorders of the kidneys

The almond tree is a native of the warmer parts of western Asia and North Africa, but it has been extensively distributed all over the warm temperate regions of the world. The tree has always been a favourite in England but mainly for its blossom. The fresh, sweet almond nut possesses demulcent and nutrient properties and this emulsion is of great use in stones, gravel or strangulation and other disorders of the kidneys, bladder and biliary ducts.

5 ounces (1 cup) blanched almonds
½ pint (1 cup) barley water (see page 22)

Chop the almonds and pound in a pestle and mortar until reduced to a paste. Then gradually stir in sufficient barley water to make the consistency slightly thicker than milk. This palatable medicine can be taken freely and you will find it brings welcome relief in any of the aforementioned conditions.

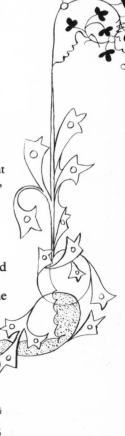

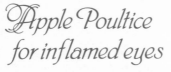

Apple Poultice
for inflamed eyes

Over the centuries the apple has acquired a universal reputation both as a preventative ("An apple a day keeps the doctor away") and as a curative food and remedy. It is full of minerals and vitamins and, taken internally, is good for many diverse ailments as wide-ranging as constipation, rheumatism, gout, anaemia. However, here it is used as a poultice to be used externally to ease sore, inflamed eyes.

2 cooking apples
2 tablespoons water

Core the apples and chop roughly. Simmer with the water in a saucepan until really soft and mashy. Allow to cool, then put 2 spoonfuls into the centre of 2 squares of muslin or large cotton handkerchiefs. Gather up the corners and press the poultices on to the closed eyes. Lie down and relax for 10 minutes.

Eye Bath

This soothes tired or inflamed eyes, but my sister Brigid swears that the most beneficial part of the treatment is the fact that you have to lie down and relax with your eyes closed for 5 or 10 minutes.

1 teaspoon honey
1 cup water

Add the honey to the water and bring to the boil. Simmer for 5 minutes. Allow to cool and if you have an eye bath, bathe the eyes 2 or 3 times a day, otherwise soak pads of cotton wool in the solution and lie back with your eyes closed, place the cotton wool pads over your eyes and relax for 5 minutes or so, as recommended by Brigid.

Onion Disinfectant

It is one of the oldest beliefs that a cut onion will absorb any illness that is about and disinfect the air. It is for this reason that one should never use up half an onion that has been lying around in the kitchen for a day or two. A cut onion, placed on a saucer in a sick room will supposedly absorb all germs and disinfect the air. The onion should be replaced daily and the old one burnt or otherwise thoroughly disposed of.

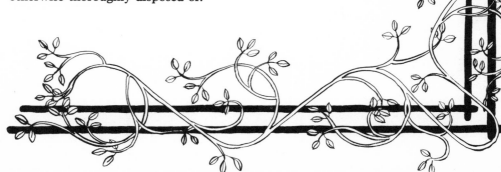

Epsom Salts Foot Bath

Epsom salts (magnesium sulphate) is so called because it was originally obtained by the evaporation of the water of a mineral spring at Epsom in Surrey (England). According to tradition, the spring was discovered in 1615 by a farmer who noticed that his cows refused to drink from this spring in spite of the prevailing drought. On analysis the water was found to contain the bitter purgative, sulphate of magnesia.
In this remedy, which comes strongly recommended by my local chemist, the epsom salts are used in a foot bath which is a very good, albeit old-fashioned, treatment for a cold.

3 pints (7½ cups) hot water
4 ounces (1 cup) Epsom salts

Fill a large bowl with water as hot as can be tolerated. Add the Epsom salts and sit in a warm place with the feet in the bath for up to 20 minutes. On removing the feet from the water, dry them well and keep warm.

To Cure Cramp

To treat a limb with cramp, the remedy is to bind fresh periwinkle around it and the cramp will disappear.

A Whitlow Remedy

This eases painful whitlows and other ailments of the fingers where the skin isn't broken. I once tried it on a scratched finger and the combination of lemon and salt on open skin had me jumping up and down, exclaiming wildly, and holding the smarting finger under running water. An experience not to be repeated. But it does work well on other swellings or inflammations of the fingers.

Take a whole lemon and heat it in the oven. Cut the top off and poke the handle of a wooden spoon down the centre. Pack this with common salt and push the affected finger inside and keep it there as long as possible. Repeat the treatment as necessary.

Garlic Plugs
to stop bleeding from the nose

Using a garlic press, squeeze the juice from 2 or 3 cloves of garlic on to a small piece of lint (or 2 if both nostrils are bleeding) which has been soaked in vinegar. Roll the lint into a plug and place it up the nostril. It makes your eyes smart but it does stop your nose bleeding.

Periwinkle
to stop bleeding of the mouth or nose

The botanical name for periwinkle, *Vinca,* means 'to bind' and alludes both to its habit of growth and also to its astringent and tonic qualities. It "stays bleeding of the mouth if chewed" and the bruised leaves, rolled and put up the nostrils will stop them bleeding. It certainly worked for my nose-bleeds when I was young but that may have been partly due to my utter surprise at having a rolled up leaf pushed up my nose.

Watercress
to prevent bleeding of the gums

Fresh, raw watercress should be chewed energetically several times a day to remedy bleeding and spongy gums.

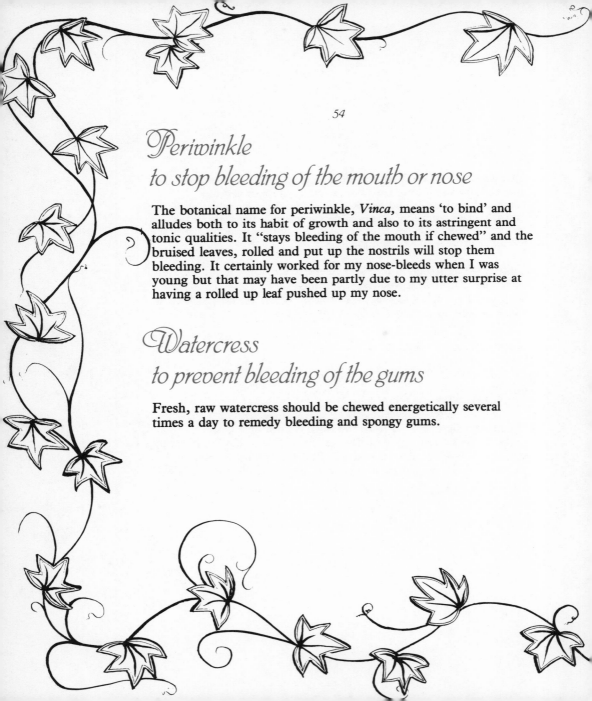

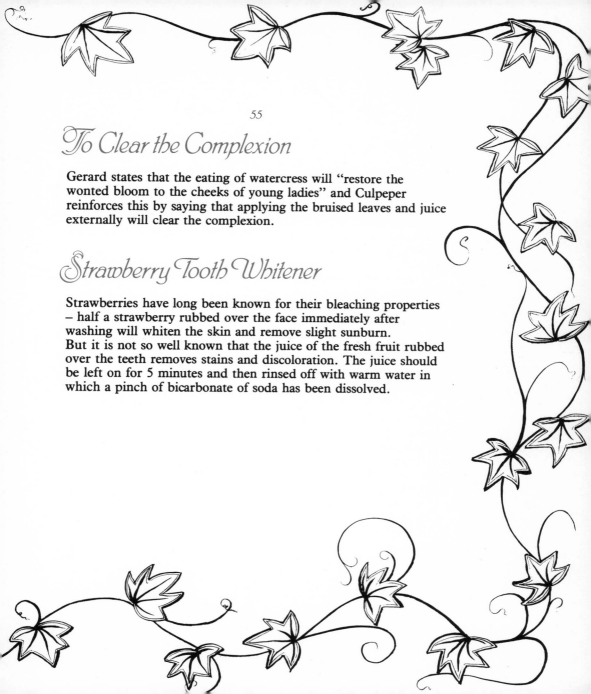

To Clear the Complexion

Gerard states that the eating of watercress will "restore the wonted bloom to the cheeks of young ladies" and Culpeper reinforces this by saying that applying the bruised leaves and juice externally will clear the complexion.

Strawberry Tooth Whitener

Strawberries have long been known for their bleaching properties – half a strawberry rubbed over the face immediately after washing will whiten the skin and remove slight sunburn.
But it is not so well known that the juice of the fresh fruit rubbed over the teeth removes stains and discoloration. The juice should be left on for 5 minutes and then rinsed off with warm water in which a pinch of bicarbonate of soda has been dissolved.

Onion
to afford relief in headache & migraine

Onions used to be taken to give considerable relief in cases of neuralgic headache or migraine. They work equally well either internally or externally, or you can combine the two by eating a boiled Spanish onion while holding an onion poultice to your head.

To make the onion poultice, the boiled onion is pressed in a sieve to remove excess moisture, then mashed with a fork and spread on to a piece of linen or muslin which is then folded over and applied, cold, to the head.

Vinegar Pack

As a child, I used to think my great uncle was slightly potty when he sat in his favourite chair with a wet hanky on his forehead. Only later did he explain that he was using a very old and simple remedy for a headache – a cloth soaked in vinegar, wrung out, folded into three and applied to the head.

I'm not sure whether it's the fumes from the vinegar or the tightening effect of it on the forehead, but this certainly brings relief, but be careful not to let drips of vinegar run down into your eyes as it really does smart.

Witch Hazel
for varicose veins or a black eye

Witch hazel has long been used by the North American Indians as poultices for painful swellings and tumours.

You can buy extract of, or distilled, witch hazel from the chemist or drugstore. A lint bandage soaked in this and bound around varicose veins brings relief and reduces the swelling and constriction.

A similar treatment is good for a black eye – soak a piece of lint in extract of witch hazel, bind it over the closed eye and keep the bandage moist.

For both these remedies it is preferable if you can lie down with your feet slightly raised.

To Remove Warts

Apply the milky juice of the freshly-broken stalk of a fig to the wart. A slightly inflamed area will appear around the wart which will eventually shrivel and fall off.

Similarly, the juice from the stalk of a dandelion flower, if applied liberally during a period of 4-5 days, will also do away with the wart.

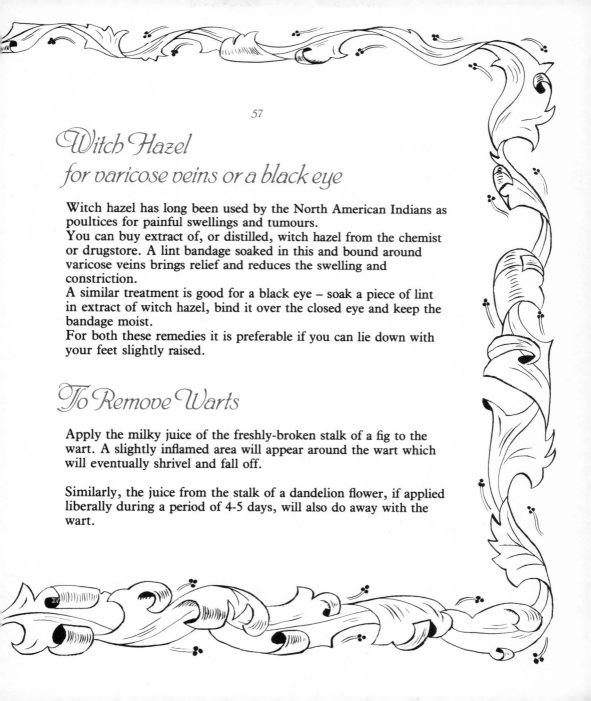

To Cure Hiccups

When any of his children had hiccups, my father used to put his hand into his pocket and pull out a handful of loose change and say "If you can hiccup once more, you can have all this." It worked without fail every time – we never could summon up another single hiccup. We always ended up ruefully thinking how much richer we would have been if only we could have.
Now that I've left home I use this much less exciting method to cure an attack of hiccups.
The remedy is to take a lump of sugar saturated with fresh lemon juice and let it slowly dissolve in the mouth. If necessary the treatment can be repeated but I find I hardly ever need more than 2 or 3 doses. If you don't have any lemons available, vinegar works almost as well.

Cure for Stammering

Having never had a stammer I cannot personally vouch for this cure but it sounds feasible and well worth trying – if one has the patience . . . This is Mrs. Beeton's suggestion.

"Where there is no malformation of the organs of articulation, stammering may be remedied by reading aloud with the teeth closed. This should be practised for two hours a day, for three or four months."

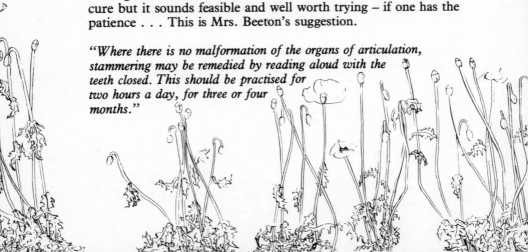

To Cure a Corn

Everyone has their favourite cure for corns and old books can suggest a dozen more, but I have only listed a small selection of my favourite ones.

Lay a sliver of fresh garlic on the affected spot and bind it with a plaster or bandage. Renew the garlic daily and after about 8 days the corn will drop off.

Wrap a strip of pineapple peel around the corn, repeating the treatment daily for about 6 days until the corn disappears.

A slice of lemon bound on overnight will work wonders before morning.

The acrid, orange-coloured juice of the greater celandine, used fresh, cures corns as well as warts, but should not be allowed to touch any other part of the skin as it will cause irritation.

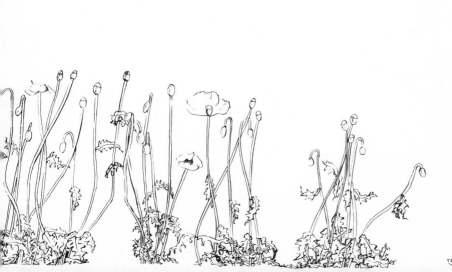
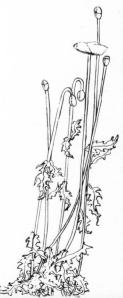

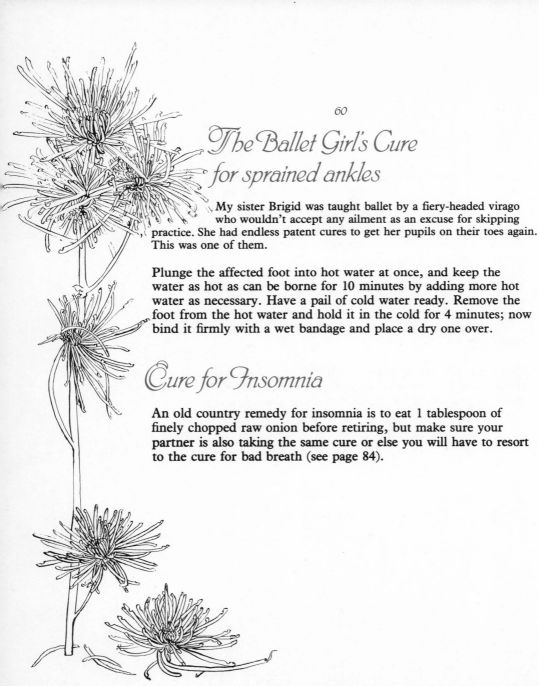

The Ballet Girl's Cure
for sprained ankles

My sister Brigid was taught ballet by a fiery-headed virago who wouldn't accept any ailment as an excuse for skipping practice. She had endless patent cures to get her pupils on their toes again. This was one of them.

Plunge the affected foot into hot water at once, and keep the water as hot as can be borne for 10 minutes by adding more hot water as necessary. Have a pail of cold water ready. Remove the foot from the hot water and hold it in the cold for 4 minutes; now bind it firmly with a wet bandage and place a dry one over.

Cure for Insomnia

An old country remedy for insomnia is to eat 1 tablespoon of finely chopped raw onion before retiring, but make sure your partner is also taking the same cure or else you will have to resort to the cure for bad breath (see page 84).

Infusion of Cardamoms for indigestion

Cardamoms are expensive – but they are little gems. They are greenish-grey, plump ovoid fruits which contain small black seeds in three cell like structures. They have a strong aromatic smell and taste warm, spicy and sweet.
The seeds alone can be chewed to cure an upset stomach and they are also good for headaches. This infusion is an easy, tasty way of taking advantage of all the carminative and digestive properties of this spice.

½ pint (1¼ pints) water
1 ounce (⅓ cup) cardamoms
½-1 teaspoon honey

Bring the water to the boil, add the cardamoms and simmer for 10 minutes. Stir in sufficient honey to taste and take a small glassful of this infusion, warm, before and after meals.

Heartburn Antidote

Cases of heartburn can often be immediately relieved by eating 6 or 8 blanched, sweet almonds. They *must* be well chewed before swallowing otherwise they will just increase your general discomfort.

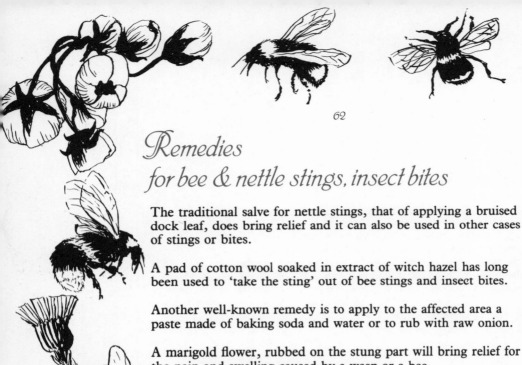

Remedies
for bee & nettle stings, insect bites

The traditional salve for nettle stings, that of applying a bruised dock leaf, does bring relief and it can also be used in other cases of stings or bites.

A pad of cotton wool soaked in extract of witch hazel has long been used to 'take the sting' out of bee stings and insect bites.

Another well-known remedy is to apply to the affected area a paste made of baking soda and water or to rub with raw onion.

A marigold flower, rubbed on the stung part will bring relief for the pain and swelling caused by a wasp or a bee.

A bruised plantain leaf will similarly ease the irritation.

Another Freckle Remover

Pliny said that "A liniment made with cress applied with vinegar, taketh off all spots and freckles of the visage." It is probable that he was referring to watercress, not cress of mustard and cress fame, though that may work equally well.

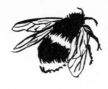

Buttermilk Freckle Bleach

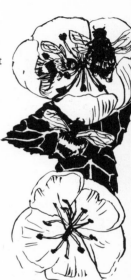

Personally, I like freckles and think them most attractive but there are others who disagree – and this mixture can also be used to effect on age spots and other similar skin discolorations. This is a very mild bleach but before applying it to the face lightly oil the skin with almond or similar light oil.

6 tablespoons buttermilk
1 teaspoon grated fresh horseradish

Combine the ingredients and apply to the ready-oiled skin that is to be treated. Leave on for 20 minutes then wash off with warm water. If it has been used on the face, moisturize after rinsing.

Dandelion Freckle Bleach

Regular washing with this lotion will gradually fade freckles

1 cup freshly opened dandelion flowers
1½ cups (3¾ cups) water

Add the dandelion flowers to the water and bring to the boil. Simmer for 30 minutes then strain through a sieve lined with muslin. Use to wash the face night and morning and watch the freckles fade.

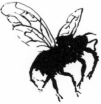

Anti-wrinkle Lotion

Glycerine and honey are two of the oldest moisturizers known. This is a smooth, delicately perfumed lotion that is easy and pleasant to use, if a bit sticky.

1 tablespoon glycerine
1 tablespoon rosewater
1 tablespoon witch hazel
3 tablespoons clear honey

Mix all the ingredients thoroughly and store in a screw-topped jar. Apply to the clean face and neck, night and morning.

Dairymaid's Lotion for chapped hands

Have you ever noticed how dairymaids always seem to have soft, smooth hands? If you massage this lotion into your hands twice a day you too will soon have hands like a dairymaid.

1 slice of lemon
½ cup milk

Put the lemon in the milk and leave for 2-3 hours until the milk has curdled slightly. Remove the lemon and use the lotion whenever necessary. Keep it in the refrigerator or else it will go completely sour and unpleasant. As it is, it has the consistency of thick cream and smells of lemons and is quite pleasant to use, if a bit runny and wet.

Cucumber Lotion for chapped hands

It is a lovely light green, fresh-smelling lotion that rubs in easily and leaves the hands soft, smooth and sweetly scented.
When cucumbers are cheap and plentiful in the summer, I make up large quantities of this delightful lotion and use it liberally after baths as a body lotion. It is particularly light and refreshing in hot weather.

2-inch piece of cucumber, peeled
1 tablespoon witch hazel extract
1 teaspoon glycerine
1 teaspoon rosewater

Chop and mash the cucumber. Add the witch hazel, glycerine and rosewater. Or alternatively, all the ingredients can be put in an electric blender and whizzed up together for about 30 seconds. Bottle in a handy, plastic bottle and keep easily available so you can use it frequently, particularly after immersing the hands in water.

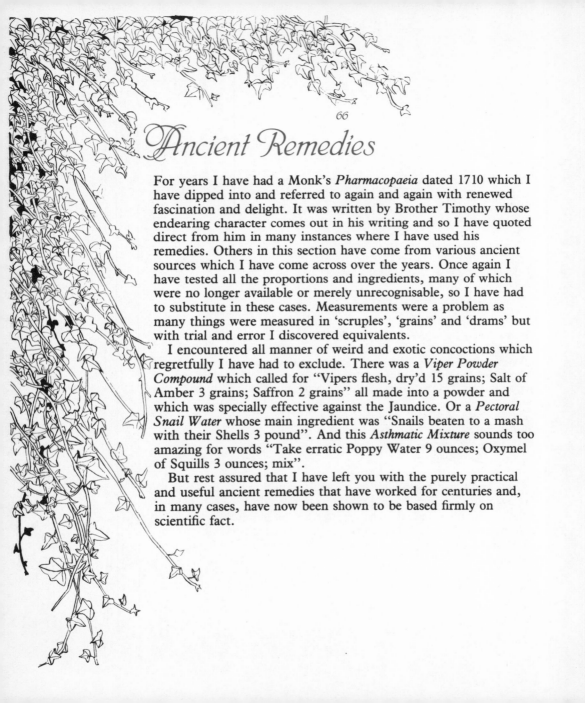

Ancient Remedies

For years I have had a Monk's *Pharmacopaeia* dated 1710 which I have dipped into and referred to again and again with renewed fascination and delight. It was written by Brother Timothy whose endearing character comes out in his writing and so I have quoted direct from him in many instances where I have used his remedies. Others in this section have come from various ancient sources which I have come across over the years. Once again I have tested all the proportions and ingredients, many of which were no longer available or merely unrecognisable, so I have had to substitute in these cases. Measurements were a problem as many things were measured in 'scruples', 'grains' and 'drams' but with trial and error I discovered equivalents.

I encountered all manner of weird and exotic concoctions which regretfully I have had to exclude. There was a *Viper Powder Compound* which called for "Vipers flesh, dry'd 15 grains; Salt of Amber 3 grains; Saffron 2 grains" all made into a powder and which was specially effective against the Jaundice. Or a *Pectoral Snail Water* whose main ingredient was "Snails beaten to a mash with their Shells 3 pound". And this *Asthmatic Mixture* sounds too amazing for words "Take erratic Poppy Water 9 ounces; Oxymel of Squills 3 ounces; mix".

But rest assured that I have left you with the purely practical and useful ancient remedies that have worked for centuries and, in many cases, have now been shown to be based firmly on scientific fact.

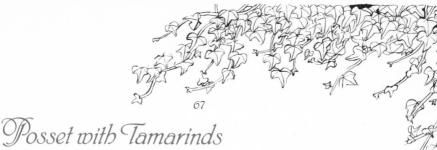

Posset with Tamarinds

The popularity of possets in olden days was probably due partly to the fact that they were heavily laced with ale or wine, which actually slightly curdled the milk and gave it a thicker consistency – all of which, together with a flavouring of spices, made an ideal remedy for colds and flu.

This posset which is good for all disorders of the stomach or bowel, relies on the acidity of the tamarinds to both curdle the milk and to flavour it.

It is interesting to know that tamarind is the acid pulp found in the pendulous, leguminous fruits of a large tropical tree that grows in India, parts of Africa and the West Indies. The tamarinds are either imported in a syrup, the outer shell of the fruit having been removed, or else in a black, rather sticky mass of seeds.

1 teaspoon tamarind pulp
½ pint (¼ cup) milk

Crush the tamarind paste with a pestle and mortar, adding a little milk to make it smooth. Heat the rest of the milk to just below boiling point. Put the tamarind paste into a bowl and quickly stir in the hot milk. Strain the mixture through a sieve and the resulting posset can be taken as often as required throughout the day. If you use too much tamarind the milk curdles completely and separates into rubbery little clots of curd and whey. If this happens during preparation the tamarind whey can be strained off and taken instead as it has equally beneficial effects and in fact is recommended in cases of fever or raised temperature.

A Decoction of Tamarinds

"It is proper for constant drink in those fevers that bring with them costiveness, drought and parching heat."

1 ounce (¼ cup) tamarinds
2 ounces (⅓ cup) raisins, stoned
1½ pints (3¾ cups) water

Boil the tamarinds and raisins in the water until the liquid is reduced by one-third. Strain, and drink this milky-brown liquid hot. It has a warm, wholesome aroma of raisins and, as tamarinds contain citric acid, this makes a most refreshing drink that will reduce fevers.

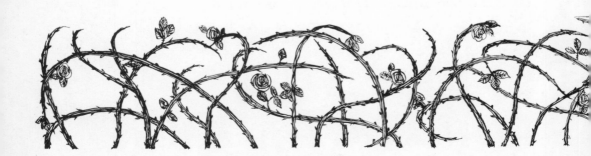

A Consolating Mixture

This recipe comes from an ancient monk's pharmacopoeia which I have had for years. The mixture is utterly delicious and gives you a warm glow – as the monk himself says: "It's proper for such only as are cold, weak and languishing. I should by no means advise it to any of a strong and hot constitution. Let 2 tablespons be allowed night and morn, whensoever failure of spirits make it needful"

¼ pint (⅔ cup) strong cinnamon water (see page 70)
2 ounces (¼ cup) sugar
½ pint (2½ cups) dry sherry
5 tablespoons rosewater
4 drops oil of nutmeg

Heat the cinnamon water over a gentle heat, add the sugar and stir until dissolved. Remove from the heat, add the sherry, rosewater and oil of nutmeg. Take great care dropping the oil of nutmeg in as it is extremely strong and too much would completely spoil the whole mixture.

Brother Timothy, the monk who wrote the pharmacopoeia in 1710, tells how he obtained this recipe: "This medicine I fish'd out of a very worthy gentleman, in whose family it had been kept as a great secret, and was religiously delivered down, from mother to daughter, in a constant succession of several generations."

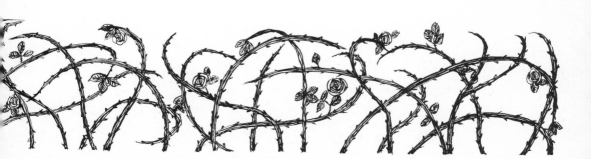

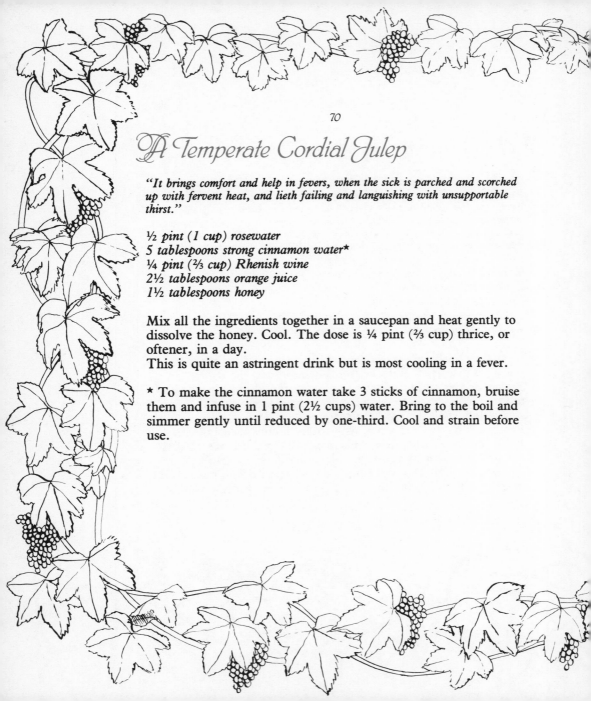

A Temperate Cordial Julep

"It brings comfort and help in fevers, when the sick is parched and scorched up with fervent heat, and lieth failing and languishing with unsupportable thirst."

½ pint (1 cup) rosewater
5 tablespoons strong cinnamon water★
¼ pint (⅔ cup) Rhenish wine
2½ tablespoons orange juice
1½ tablespoons honey

Mix all the ingredients together in a saucepan and heat gently to dissolve the honey. Cool. The dose is ¼ pint (⅔ cup) thrice, or oftener, in a day.
This is quite an astringent drink but is most cooling in a fever.

★ To make the cinnamon water take 3 sticks of cinnamon, bruise them and infuse in 1 pint (2½ cups) water. Bring to the boil and simmer gently until reduced by one-third. Cool and strain before use.

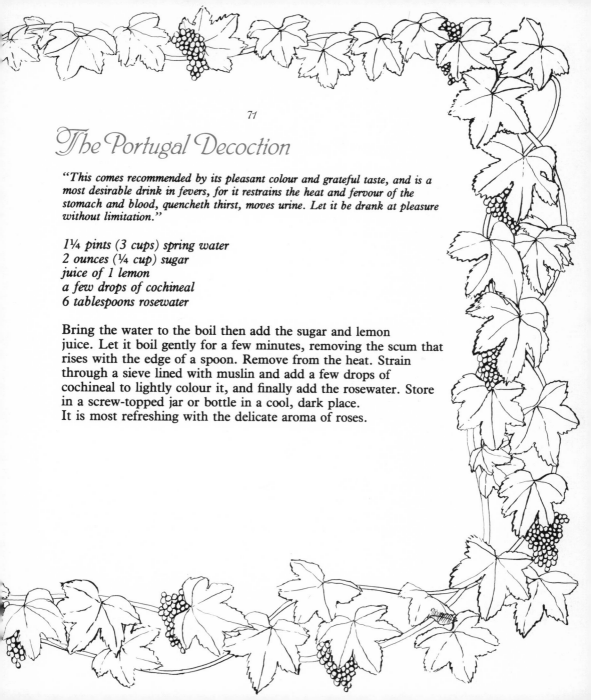

The Portugal Decoction

"This comes recommended by its pleasant colour and grateful taste, and is a most desirable drink in fevers, for it restrains the heat and fervour of the stomach and blood, quencheth thirst, moves urine. Let it be drank at pleasure without limitation."

1¼ pints (3 cups) spring water
2 ounces (¼ cup) sugar
juice of 1 lemon
a few drops of cochineal
6 tablespoons rosewater

Bring the water to the boil then add the sugar and lemon juice. Let it boil gently for a few minutes, removing the scum that rises with the edge of a spoon. Remove from the heat. Strain through a sieve lined with muslin and add a few drops of cochineal to lightly colour it, and finally add the rosewater. Store in a screw-topped jar or bottle in a cool, dark place.
It is most refreshing with the delicate aroma of roses.

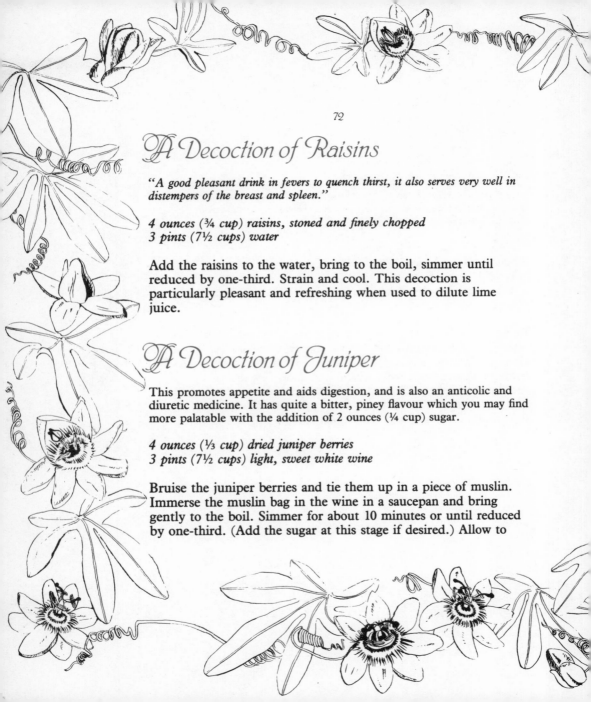

A Decoction of Raisins

"A good pleasant drink in fevers to quench thirst, it also serves very well in distempers of the breast and spleen."

4 ounces (¾ cup) raisins, stoned and finely chopped
3 pints (7½ cups) water

Add the raisins to the water, bring to the boil, simmer until reduced by one-third. Strain and cool. This decoction is particularly pleasant and refreshing when used to dilute lime juice.

A Decoction of Juniper

This promotes appetite and aids digestion, and is also an anticolic and diuretic medicine. It has quite a bitter, piney flavour which you may find more palatable with the addition of 2 ounces (¼ cup) sugar.

4 ounces (⅓ cup) dried juniper berries
3 pints (7½ cups) light, sweet white wine

Bruise the juniper berries and tie them up in a piece of muslin. Immerse the muslin bag in the wine in a saucepan and bring gently to the boil. Simmer for about 10 minutes or until reduced by one-third. (Add the sugar at this stage if desired.) Allow to

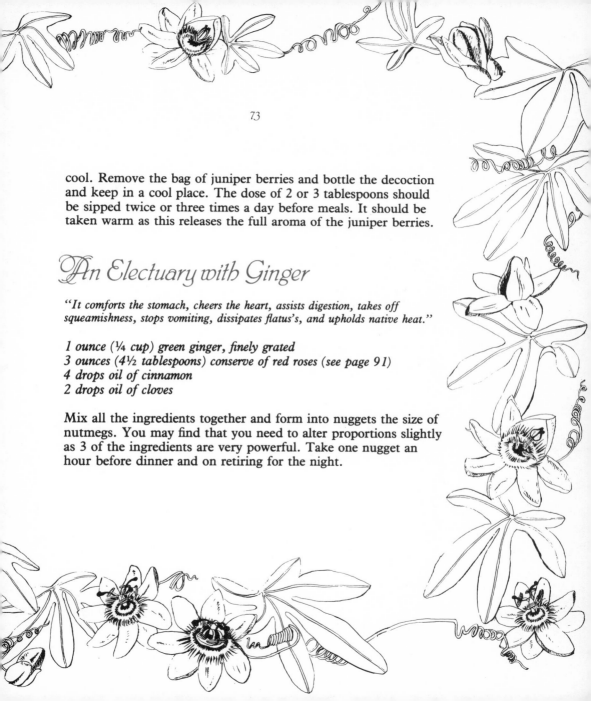

cool. Remove the bag of juniper berries and bottle the decoction and keep in a cool place. The dose of 2 or 3 tablespoons should be sipped twice or three times a day before meals. It should be taken warm as this releases the full aroma of the juniper berries.

An Electuary with Ginger

"It comforts the stomach, cheers the heart, assists digestion, takes off squeamishness, stops vomiting, dissipates flatus's, and upholds native heat."

1 ounce (¼ cup) green ginger, finely grated
3 ounces (4½ tablespoons) conserve of red roses (see page 91)
4 drops oil of cinnamon
2 drops oil of cloves

Mix all the ingredients together and form into nuggets the size of nutmegs. You may find that you need to alter proportions slightly as 3 of the ingredients are very powerful. Take one nugget an hour before dinner and on retiring for the night.

A Julep of Propriety

"To excite an appetite, take off nauseousness, and assist digestion, drink a small cupful half an hour before, and immediately after dinner daily."

½ pint (1¼ cups) white wine
5 tablespoons mint water★
4 cloves
½ ounce (½ cup) candied angelica, chopped

Heat the wine, mint water, cloves and angelica over very low heat, without boiling, for 2 hours. Remove from the heat, strain, cool and bottle. Keep in a cool, dark place and use as required.

★To make the mint water take a handful of fresh mint leaves and stalks, bruise them and infuse in ½ pint (1¼ cups) water. Leave in a warm place for 24 hours, strain and use.

Asthma Inhalant

The fumes of burning dried nettle leaves, if inhaled, will relieve bronchial and asthmatic troubles.

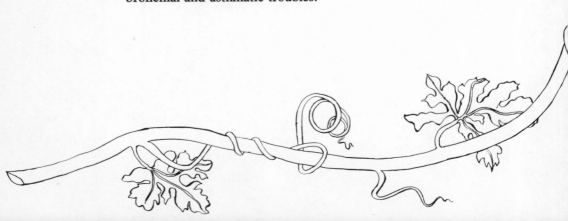

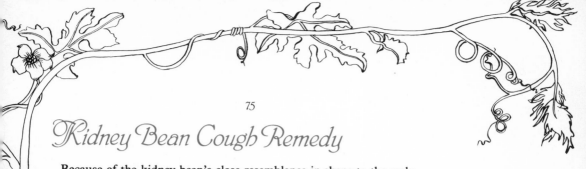

Kidney Bean Cough Remedy

Because of the kidney bean's close resemblance in shape to the male testicle, the Egyptians made it an object of sacred worship and forbad its use as a food. It is not down on record what they felt about it being used for its medicinal properties.

7 ounces (1 cup) kidney beans
2-3 cloves garlic, peeled & chopped
¾ pint (2 cups) water

Rinse the kidney beans and soak them overnight in water. Drain, and bruise them by tying them up in a clean cloth and hitting them with a rolling pin. Place the bruised beans in a saucepan with the garlic and water. Bring to the boil and simmer gently for 1½-2 hours until tender, adding more water if necessary. The resulting bean purée taken in tablespoon doses, has been known to cure otherwise incurable coughs so it should devastate your tickle.

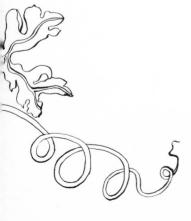

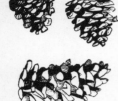

A Red Linctus

"This fine-coloured and pleasant-tasting linctus eases the throat when parched and rough and soothes a most violent cough."

½ ounce (1 tablespoon) rose-hip syrup (see page 93)
1½ tablespoons elderberry syrup (see page 92)
1½ tablespoons sweet almond oil

Mix all the ingredients together and administer 1 or 2 teaspoonfuls 3 times a day.

Ancient Cough Mixture

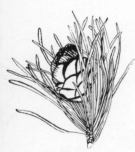

This eases the congestion and soothes the throat and altogether is an admirable remedy for persistent coughs. I always use this rather any proprietary cough mixture.

3 tablespoons clear honey
¼ pint (⅔ cup) warm water
1 tablespoon cider vinegar

Dissolve the honey in the water then mix in the vinegar. The dose is 1 teaspoon 5 or 6 times a day.

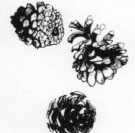

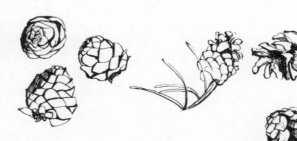

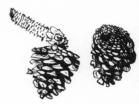

The Spanish Infusion

"When molested with a vexatious cough in the evening, take half a pint (1 cup) cold, just at going to bed. In feverish conditions with shiverings and flushes, heaviness of the head; let it be sipped off hot all day long at times, and let the patient keep himself up in his chamber to avoid the cold air."

3 pints (7½ cups) spring water
1 tablespoon cream of tartar
a pinch of saffron
8-inch piece of liquorice root

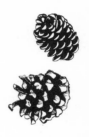

Combine all the ingredients and leave in a warm place for 24 hours to infuse. Strain and use as required.

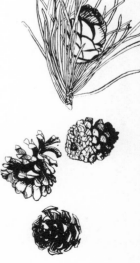

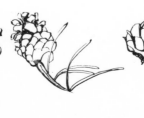

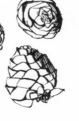

A Pectoral Decoction

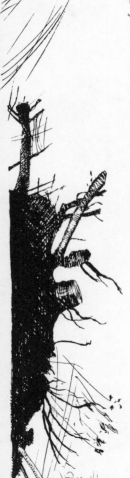

"It is endow'd with a mucilaginous, soft and friendly sweetness . . . and gives mighty relief in a cough."

1 ounce (2 tablespoons) pearl barley
1 ounce (3 tablespoons) stoned raisins
8 figs
8 dates
4-inch piece of liquorice root
3 pints (7½ cups) water
a few drops of aniseed

Add the pearl barley, raisins, figs, dates and liquorice to the water in a saucepan and bring gently to the boil. Simmer for 20 minutes until reduced by one-third, then stir in the aniseed. Allow to cool. Strain through a sieve lined with muslin and bottle. Store in a cool place. The dose may be 3 or 4 tablespoons taken 2 or 3 times a day.

A Draught for a Catarrh

For this you will need coltsfoot water which is prepared as follows: Take a handful of dried flowers or leaves of the coltsfoot and soak in 1 pint (2½ cups) of cold water for 5 minutes. Bring to the boil then allow to cool. Strain through a sieve lined with fine muslin to eliminate the down which would be an irritant.

2 egg yolks
1 tablespoon honey
½ pint (1 cup) coltsfoot water

Beat the egg yolks well, then gradually add the honey and finally the coltsfoot water, still beating well. Place in a bowl over a saucepan of gently boiling water and heat, stirring, until the mixture thickens. Give to the patient just as he goes to bed.

To describe the qualities of the soothing draught I quote direct from the pharmacopaeia:
"This draught usually gives great relief in a (let me call it) guttural, rheumatic and evening cough, caused by catching cold, which is pretty quiet all day, but returns at night, especially when one lies down in bed, incessantly disturbing, and vexatiously hindering rest. For by reason of its sweet unctuous mucilage, it so defends the larynx, that it feels not the pricking of the sharp irritating serum, and so staves off the cough, and dallies away the hour, 'till at length, the time of coughing is slipp'd, and sleep steals on."

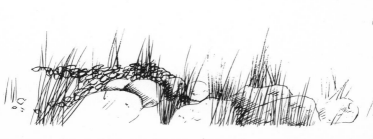

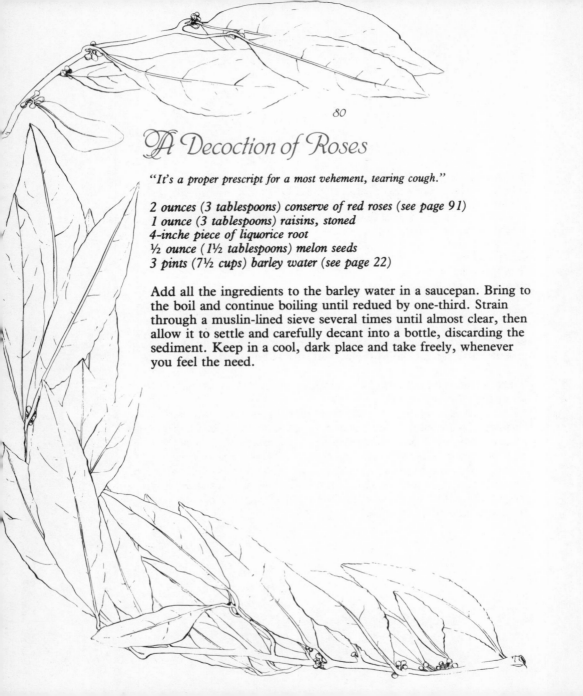

A Decoction of Roses

"It's a proper prescript for a most vehement, tearing cough."

2 ounces (3 tablespoons) conserve of red roses (see page 91)
1 ounce (3 tablespoons) raisins, stoned
4-inche piece of liquorice root
½ ounce (1½ tablespoons) melon seeds
3 pints (7½ cups) barley water (see page 22)

Add all the ingredients to the barley water in a saucepan. Bring to the boil and continue boiling until redued by one-third. Strain through a muslin-lined sieve several times until almost clear, then allow it to settle and carefully decant into a bottle, discarding the sediment. Keep in a cool, dark place and take freely, whenever you feel the need.

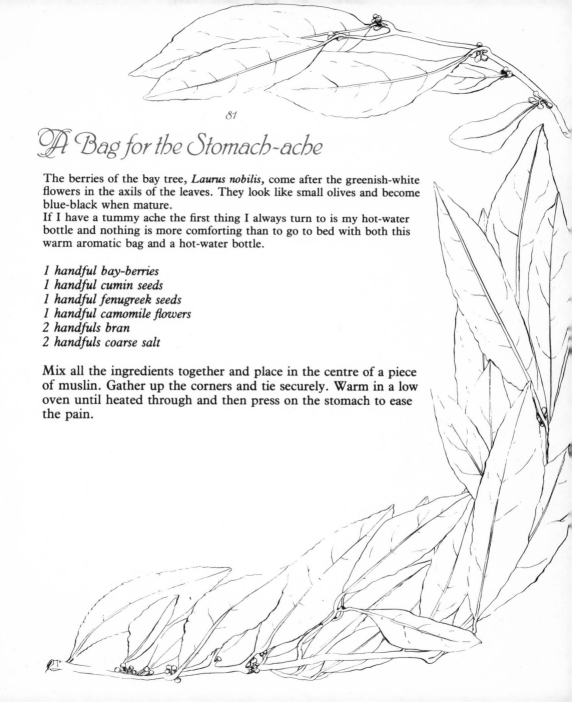

A Bag for the Stomach-ache

The berries of the bay tree, *Laurus nobilis,* come after the greenish-white flowers in the axils of the leaves. They look like small olives and become blue-black when mature.

If I have a tummy ache the first thing I always turn to is my hot-water bottle and nothing is more comforting than to go to bed with both this warm aromatic bag and a hot-water bottle.

1 handful bay-berries
1 handful cumin seeds
1 handful fenugreek seeds
1 handful camomile flowers
2 handfuls bran
2 handfuls coarse salt

Mix all the ingredients together and place in the centre of a piece of muslin. Gather up the corners and tie securely. Warm in a low oven until heated through and then press on the stomach to ease the pain.

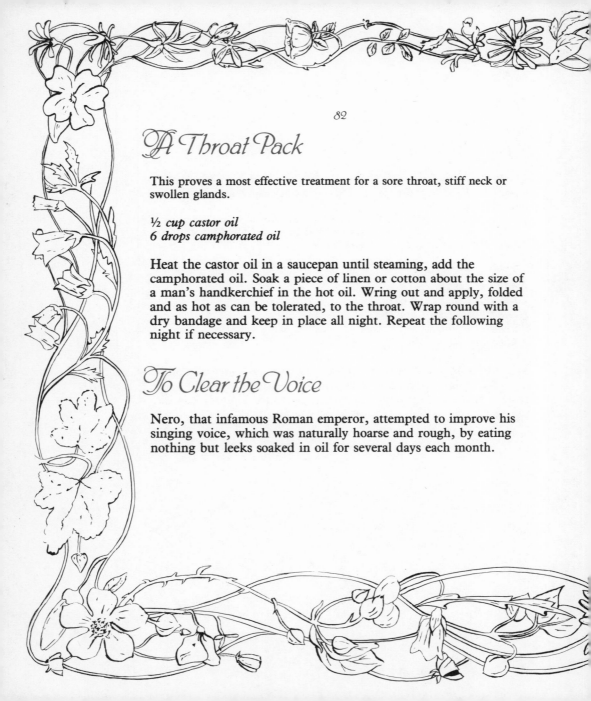

A Throat Pack

This proves a most effective treatment for a sore throat, stiff neck or swollen glands.

½ cup castor oil
6 drops camphorated oil

Heat the castor oil in a saucepan until steaming, add the camphorated oil. Soak a piece of linen or cotton about the size of a man's handkerchief in the hot oil. Wring out and apply, folded and as hot as can be tolerated, to the throat. Wrap round with a dry bandage and keep in place all night. Repeat the following night if necessary.

To Clear the Voice

Nero, that infamous Roman emperor, attempted to improve his singing voice, which was naturally hoarse and rough, by eating nothing but leeks soaked in oil for several days each month.

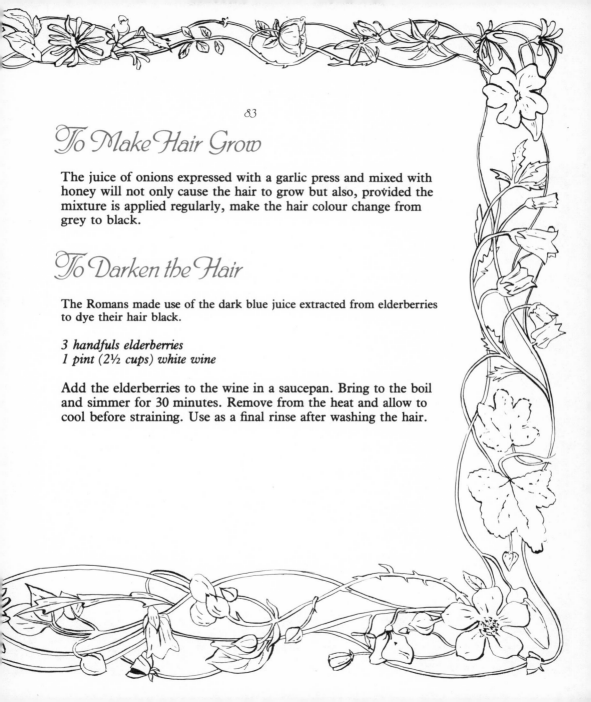

To Make Hair Grow

The juice of onions expressed with a garlic press and mixed with honey will not only cause the hair to grow but also, provided the mixture is applied regularly, make the hair colour change from grey to black.

To Darken the Hair

The Romans made use of the dark blue juice extracted from elderberries to dye their hair black.

3 handfuls elderberries
1 pint (2½ cups) white wine

Add the elderberries to the wine in a saucepan. Bring to the boil and simmer for 30 minutes. Remove from the heat and allow to cool before straining. Use as a final rinse after washing the hair.

Culpeper's Cure
for bad breath

Culpeper tells us that the juice of the red beetroot when "snuffed up the nose, helps a stinking breath".

Chewing a sprig of parsley or a few coriander seeds also sweetens the breath. Parsley is even able to mask the smell of garlic, but if you aren't careful you're then left with little bits of green all over your teeth.

Rosemary
for weakness of the brain

Rosemary has long held an important place in the cottage herb garden. It had a reputation for strengthening the memory and thus became the emblem for remembrance, friendship and a sign of fidelity between lovers.

An ancient remedy against weakness of the brain and coldness thereof was to simmer a bunch of fresh rosemary in wine and let the patient inhale the stream through the nose, keeping his head warm all the time.

Doctor Bartie's Medicine for aches & swellings

I haven't been able to discover just who Dr Bartie was but he is quoted as an authority in *The Good Hus-wives Jewell* (1597).

"Take flowers of camomile and rose leaves, steep them in white wine, making a plaister thereof, lay it on the place where any pain, ache or swelling is."

Another Headache Remedy

Take fresh green elder leaves, heat them between two plates in the oven and apply to the head. This will promptly relieve a nervous headache.

For the Cramp

"Take of rosemary leaves and chop them very small, and sew them in fine linen, and make them into garters, and wear them night and day, lay a down pillow on your legs in the night."

To Remedy the Feet
that are sore with travailing

"Take plantain and stamp (bruise) it well and anoint your feet with the juice thereof, and the pain will ease."

Roast Turnip
for chilblains

"Roast a turnip until soft, beat it to a mash, and apply it as hot as can be endured to the part affected. Let it lie on 2 or 3 days, and repeat it 2 or 3 times."

To Break a Boil

"Take the yolk of a new-laid egg, some honey and wheat-flour, and mix it well together, and spread it on a rag, and lay it on cold."

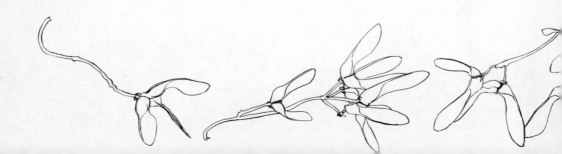

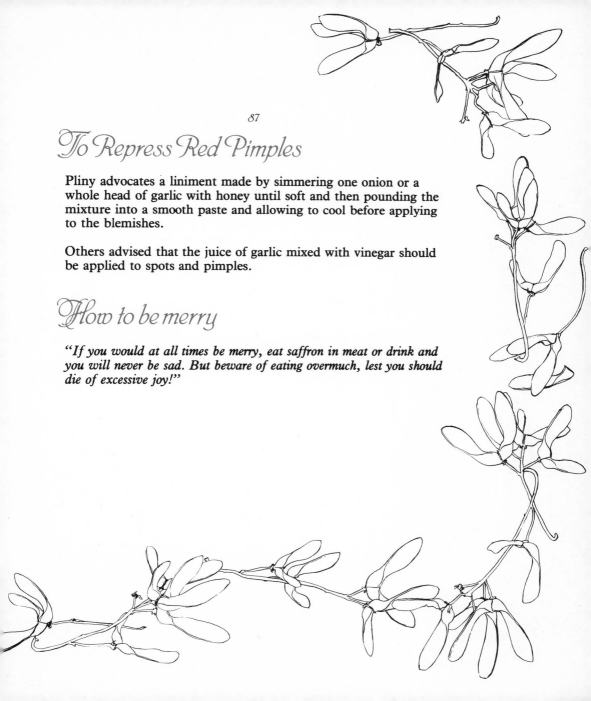

To Repress Red Pimples

Pliny advocates a liniment made by simmering one onion or a whole head of garlic with honey until soft and then pounding the mixture into a smooth paste and allowing to cool before applying to the blemishes.

Others advised that the juice of garlic mixed with vinegar should be applied to spots and pimples.

How to be merry

"If you would at all times be merry, eat saffron in meat or drink and you will never be sad. But beware of eating overmuch, lest you should die of excessive joy!"

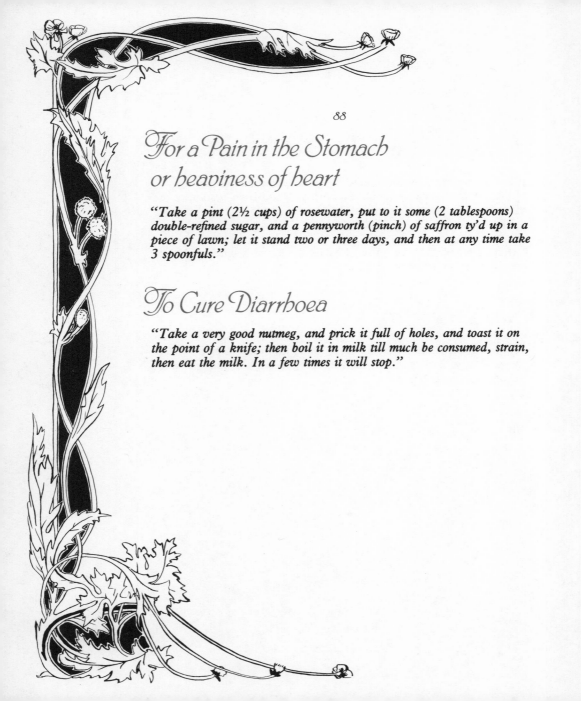

For a Pain in the Stomach or heaviness of heart

"Take a pint (2½ cups) of rosewater, put to it some (2 tablespoons) double-refined sugar, and a pennyworth (pinch) of saffron ty'd up in a piece of lawn; let it stand two or three days, and then at any time take 3 spoonfuls."

To Cure Diarrhoea

"Take a very good nutmeg, and prick it full of holes, and toast it on the point of a knife; then boil it in milk till much be consumed, strain, then eat the milk. In a few times it will stop."

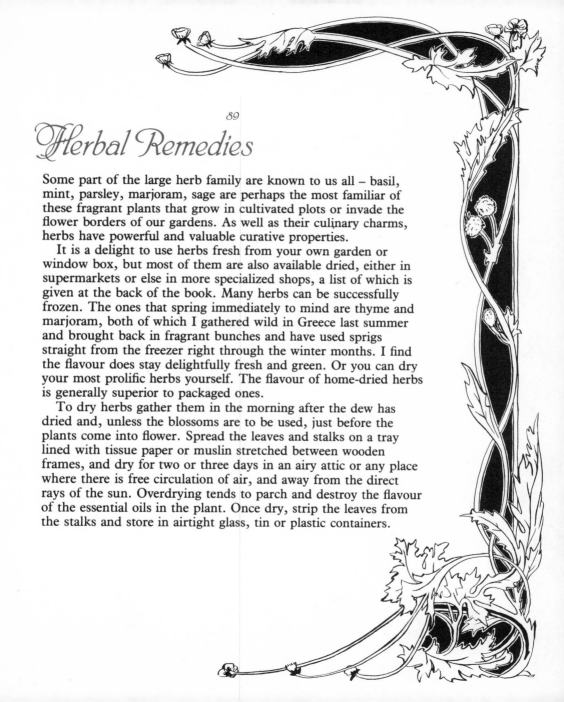

Herbal Remedies

Some part of the large herb family are known to us all – basil, mint, parsley, marjoram, sage are perhaps the most familiar of these fragrant plants that grow in cultivated plots or invade the flower borders of our gardens. As well as their culinary charms, herbs have powerful and valuable curative properties.

It is a delight to use herbs fresh from your own garden or window box, but most of them are also available dried, either in supermarkets or else in more specialized shops, a list of which is given at the back of the book. Many herbs can be successfully frozen. The ones that spring immediately to mind are thyme and marjoram, both of which I gathered wild in Greece last summer and brought back in fragrant bunches and have used sprigs straight from the freezer right through the winter months. I find the flavour does stay delightfully fresh and green. Or you can dry your most prolific herbs yourself. The flavour of home-dried herbs is generally superior to packaged ones.

To dry herbs gather them in the morning after the dew has dried and, unless the blossoms are to be used, just before the plants come into flower. Spread the leaves and stalks on a tray lined with tissue paper or muslin stretched between wooden frames, and dry for two or three days in an airy attic or any place where there is free circulation of air, and away from the direct rays of the sun. Overdrying tends to parch and destroy the flavour of the essential oils in the plant. Once dry, strip the leaves from the stalks and store in airtight glass, tin or plastic containers.

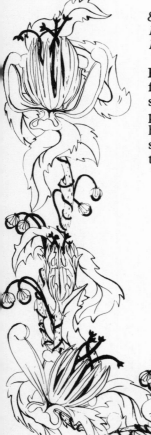

Syrup of Violets

This is an excellent gentle laxative which, when given with an equal amount of sweet almond oil, can even be given to children. The ancients held that syrup of violets could cure a variety of ailments from ague, epilepsy, inflammation of the eyes, sleeplessness to pleurisy, jaundice and quinsy.

8 ounes (3 cups) fresh sweet violet flowers
1 pint (2½ cups) boiling water
1 pound (2 cups) sugar

Pour the boiling water over the violet flowers and leave to infuse for 24 hours. Strain through a sieve lined with muslin, into a saucepan. Add the sugar and bring gently to just below boiling point, stirring to dissolve the sugar. Simmer until reduced by half, and of a syrupy consistency. The dose is ½-1 teaspoon of the syrup (with an equal amount of sweet almond oil for children) taken 3 or 4 times a day.

Conserve of Red Roses

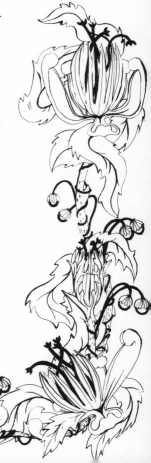

Of all the roses known, the dark red rose, *Rosa gallica,* is the one to use for medicinal purposes. The Arabs were one of the first people to realise the medical potential of roses and Avicenna tells of a consumptive who was on the point of death and then recovered his health by taking a conserve of red roses. The recipe probably hasn't altered much since then. It is essential to gather the roses on a fine day, once the dew has dried on the petals, and to snip off the lighter-coloured, lower portion of each petal before use.

8 ounces (2 cups) red rose petals
1½ pounds (3 cups) fine white sugar
rosewater

In a stone pestle and mortar pound the rose petals with the sugar. Add sufficient rosewater to make it the consistency of honey. Store in a tightly stoppered jar in a cool dark place.

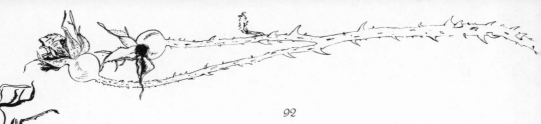

Elderberry Syrup

To make this lovely syrup, take the stems off as many elderberries as you have collected. Put them into a large saucepan and crush them with a weight or a large wooden spoon. Heat gently until the juice flows out, then simmer, covered, for 15 minutes. Remove from the heat and strain, pressing through as much juice as possible. Measure the juice and for each ½ pint (1¼ cups) of juice allow 8 ounces (1 cup) sugar and 1 tablespoon lemon juice. Bring to the boil, stirring constantly. Boil for about 10 minutes until the liquid has reduced by about one-third and is of a syrupy consistency. Bottle in clean, dry bottles and use frequently – diluted for children's drinks or summer cordials and also in the preparation of the fine Red Linctus for coughs (see page 76).

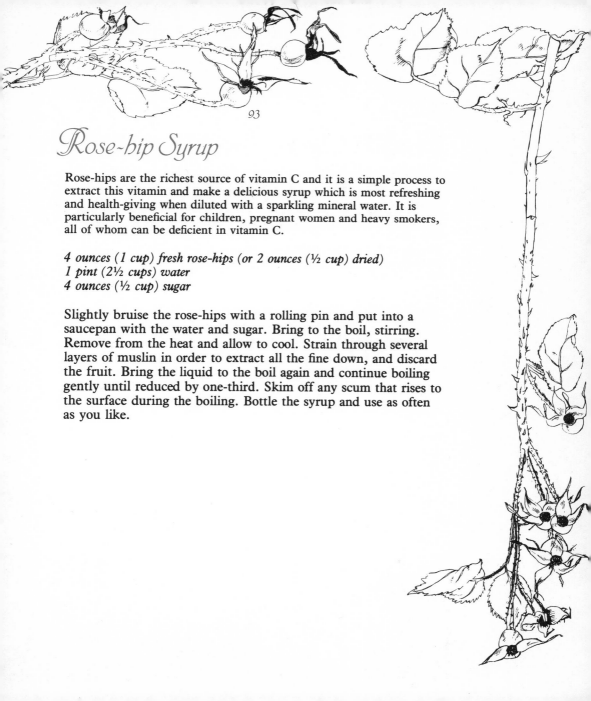

Rose-hip Syrup

Rose-hips are the richest source of vitamin C and it is a simple process to extract this vitamin and make a delicious syrup which is most refreshing and health-giving when diluted with a sparkling mineral water. It is particularly beneficial for children, pregnant women and heavy smokers, all of whom can be deficient in vitamin C.

4 ounces (1 cup) fresh rose-hips (or 2 ounces (½ cup) dried)
1 pint (2½ cups) water
4 ounces (½ cup) sugar

Slightly bruise the rose-hips with a rolling pin and put into a saucepan with the water and sugar. Bring to the boil, stirring. Remove from the heat and allow to cool. Strain through several layers of muslin in order to extract all the fine down, and discard the fruit. Bring the liquid to the boil again and continue boiling gently until reduced by one-third. Skim off any scum that rises to the surface during the boiling. Bottle the syrup and use as often as you like.

Chickweed Water
for weight loss

Chickweed water is also useful in cases of constipation which may explain why it is a firmly held old wives' belief that drinking this freely does help weight loss.
I have tried it and find it rather lacking in flavour without the addition of lemon juice and . . . honey, which rather defeats the purpose of taking it for losing weight.

1 pint (2½ cups) boiling water
1 handful fresh chickweed

Pour the boiling water over the chickweed and allow to stand for 10 minutes. Strain and take freely throughout the day.

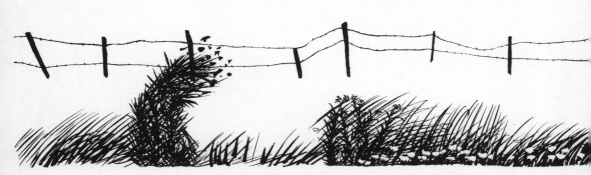

Elderflower Water

Elderflower water was an essential addition to every lady's dressing table as it was used to clear the complexion, remove freckles, allay the effect of sunburn and keep the skin soft and white. I try to always take a bottle of this with me on summer holidays as it is a refreshing, soothing lotion for sun or wind burnt skin.

Remove the stalks from a sufficient quantity of elderflowers to fill a large earthenware jar. Pack the flowers in well then pour on 4 pints (10 cups) of boiling water. When slightly cooled add 3 tablespoons of pure alcohol or rectified spirits. Cover the jar with a folded cloth and leave in a warm place for 6 hours before moving it to a cool place to become quite cold. Strain through muslin, then bottle and cork securely. Use this lotion freely on the face, neck and hands.

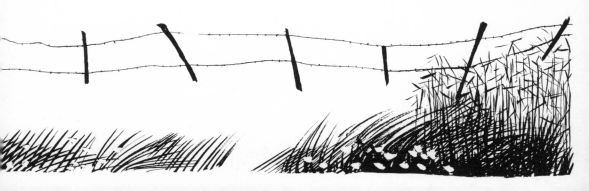

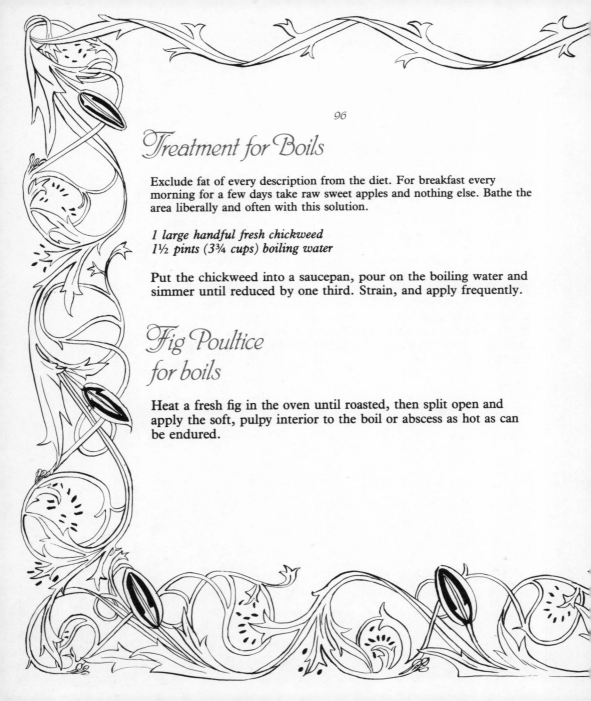

Treatment for Boils

Exclude fat of every description from the diet. For breakfast every morning for a few days take raw sweet apples and nothing else. Bathe the area liberally and often with this solution.

1 large handful fresh chickweed
1½ pints (3¾ cups) boiling water

Put the chickweed into a saucepan, pour on the boiling water and simmer until reduced by one third. Strain, and apply frequently.

Fig Poultice
for boils

Heat a fresh fig in the oven until roasted, then split open and apply the soft, pulpy interior to the boil or abscess as hot as can be endured.

Coltsfoot Decoction for asthma & coughs

The botanical name for coltsfoot, *Tussilago,* means 'cough dispeller' and the leaves can be smoked to ease a cough. Being unable to smoke anything without coughing and spluttering, I prefer to take this decoction, sweetened with honey and sometimes for a change, with a slice of lemon too.

1 handful fresh coltsfoot leaves (or 1 ounce (½ cup) dried)
2 pints (5 cups) water
honey &/or lemon to taste

Put the coltsfoot leaves in the water and bring to the boil. Simmer until reduced by half. Strain, add honey and/or lemon to taste and take small cupfuls frequently, whenever the chest feels tight and congested.

Thyme Syrup
for whooping cough

Thyme is an aromatic antiseptic, the dried flowers and stalks often being sprinkled among stored linen to preserve it fresh and free from insects. Bees love the flowers and impart the sweet flavour to their honey. Mount Hymettus, near Athens, is covered with blankets of wild thyme and consequently Hymettus honey is considered exceptional in flavour and sweetness.

This thyme syrup has been used extensively as a safe cure for whooping cough.

1 handful fresh thyme
1-2 tablespoons clear honey

Strip the leaves off the stalks of thyme and pound in a pestle and mortar. Add the honey and give a teaspoonful of this syrup as often as required to bring relief.

Camomile Tonic

In ancient times camomile was considered a sovereign remedy and was prescribed for many diverse ailments. The Egyptians dedicated it to the sun because of its effectiveness against fevers. It is an excellent tonic and an old-fashioned but extremely efficacious remedy for hysterical and nervous people.

2 ounces (1 cup) camomile flowers
1 tablespoon lemon juice
3 tablespoons honey
1½ pints (3¾ cups) white wine

Add the camomile flowers, lemon juice and honey to the white wine in a bowl. Stir well and leave, covered, in a cool, dark place for 10 days. Strain through a sieve lined with muslin and take a small glassful 3 times a day before meals.

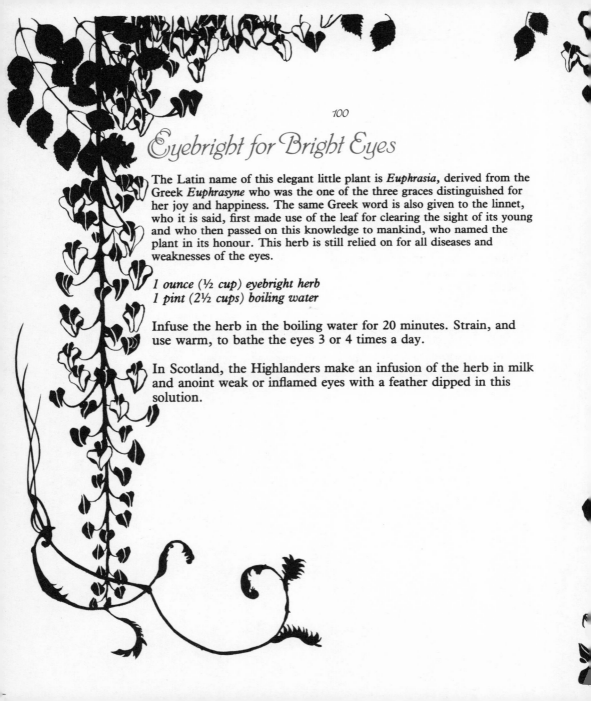

Eyebright for Bright Eyes

The Latin name of this elegant little plant is *Euphrasia,* derived from the Greek *Euphrasyne* who was the one of the three graces distinguished for her joy and happiness. The same Greek word is also given to the linnet, who it is said, first made use of the leaf for clearing the sight of its young and who then passed on this knowledge to mankind, who named the plant in its honour. This herb is still relied on for all diseases and weaknesses of the eyes.

1 ounce (½ cup) eyebright herb
1 pint (2½ cups) boiling water

Infuse the herb in the boiling water for 20 minutes. Strain, and use warm, to bathe the eyes 3 or 4 times a day.

In Scotland, the Highlanders make an infusion of the herb in milk and anoint weak or inflamed eyes with a feather dipped in this solution.

Parsley Eye Lotion

Parsley is rich in calcium, iron and vitamins and is an important herb for many purposes – here it is used as a soothing eye lotion to eliminate puffiness and to cure sties. An ancient practice to cure a stye is to rub it with a gold wedding ring. In order to effect a quick and complete cure one should perhaps use both treatments in conjunction with each other.

½ pint (1¼ cups) boiling water
1 handful fresh parsley leaves and stalks

Pour the boiling water over the parsley and leave to infuse for 10 minutes. Strain and allow to cool until tepid before soaking pads of cotton wool in the infusion and applying to the closed eyes. This is more beneficial if the patient lies down with the pads over the eyes and relaxes for at least 15 minutes.

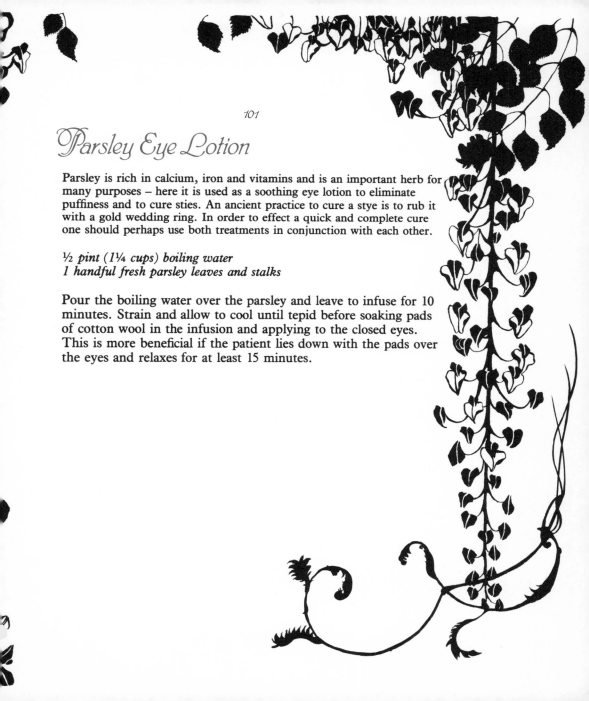

Plantain Infusion
for diarrhoea & piles

1 pint (2½ cups) boiling water
1 ounce (1 cup) fresh plantain leaves, chopped

Pour the boiling water over the chopped leaves and allow to stand
in a warm place for 20 minutes. Strain and allow to cool. Take a
small glassful 3 or 4 times a day to bring great relief for diarrhoea
and piles.

Fennel for Fleas

When fennel seeds are crushed they emit a strong, camphor-like
smell which probably explains why the powdered seeds are used
to effect to keep fleas away from kennels and stables.

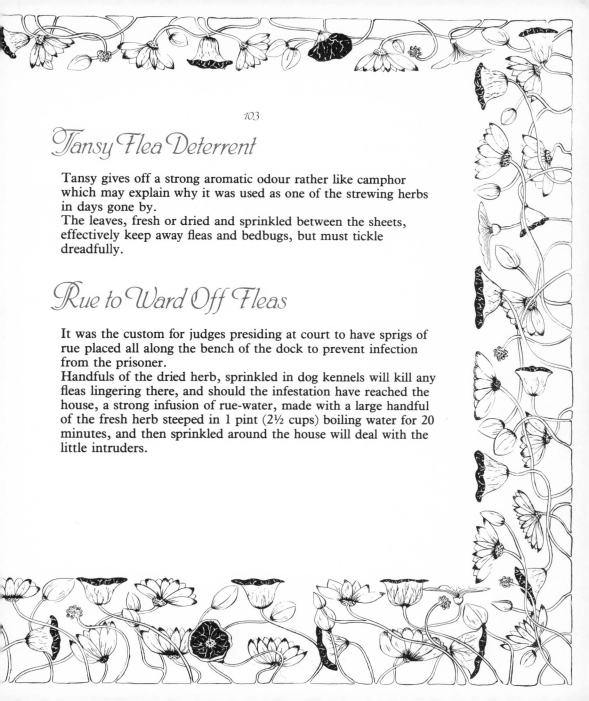

Tansy Flea Deterrent

Tansy gives off a strong aromatic odour rather like camphor which may explain why it was used as one of the strewing herbs in days gone by.

The leaves, fresh or dried and sprinkled between the sheets, effectively keep away fleas and bedbugs, but must tickle dreadfully.

Rue to Ward Off Fleas

It was the custom for judges presiding at court to have sprigs of rue placed all along the bench of the dock to prevent infection from the prisoner.

Handfuls of the dried herb, sprinkled in dog kennels will kill any fleas lingering there, and should the infestation have reached the house, a strong infusion of rue-water, made with a large handful of the fresh herb steeped in 1 pint (2½ cups) boiling water for 20 minutes, and then sprinkled around the house will deal with the little intruders.

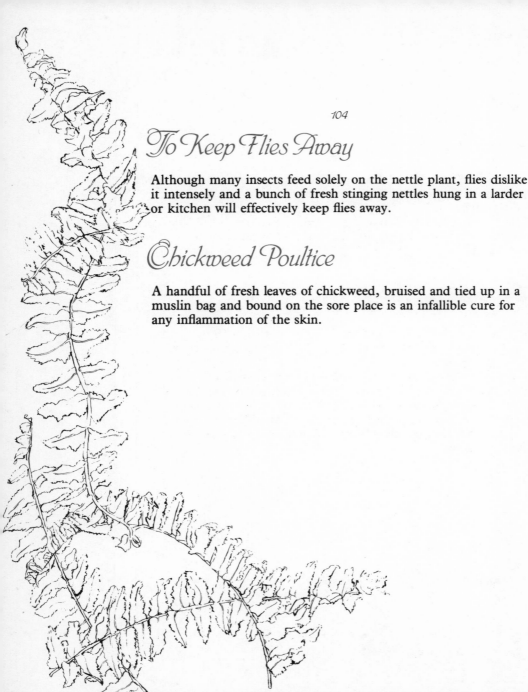

To Keep Flies Away

Although many insects feed solely on the nettle plant, flies dislike
it intensely and a bunch of fresh stinging nettles hung in a larder
or kitchen will effectively keep flies away.

Chickweed Poultice

A handful of fresh leaves of chickweed, bruised and tied up in a
muslin bag and bound on the sore place is an infallible cure for
any inflammation of the skin.

Comfrey Poultice

For thousands of years comfrey has been used to promote healings of wounds, ulcers and fractured bones. This is a soothing poultice which brings great relief to sprains and muscular aches and pains.
A friend of mine was bumped by a car recently and applied comfrey poultices all down his right hip and thigh which were severely grazed and sore. The next morning there was no bruising at all and the tissues healed remarkably well and quickly.

2 handfuls fresh comfrey leaves
1 pint (2½ cups) boiling water

Chop the comfrey leaves finely, pour the boiling water over and soak for 5 minutes. Drain, and spread the leaves on to a cloth wrung out in hot water. Fold this over and apply to the affected part. Bind with a dry bandage and renew the poultice as necessary. It is important to use fresh comfrey leaves for each new poultice, not just to reheat the old ones.

Periwinkle Ointment

This is an old-established homely remedy for all inflammatory ailments of the skin and excellent for bleeding piles.

3 handfuls fresh periwinkle leaves
4 ounces (½ cup) lard (shortening)

Bruise the periwinkle leaves and heat them gently with the lard in a saucepan. Stir and pound the mixture with a wooden spoon as it is heating. Simmer gently for 8-10 minutes. Strain through a sieve and bottle while still warm. Use as necessary for healing all minor domestic burns, scalds and inflammations of the skin.

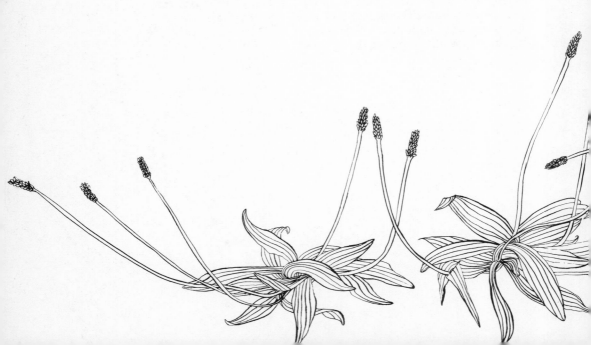

Plantain Poultice

When I was young we used to call the fruit of this familiar 'weed' soldiers and used to have great battles, striking each other's soldier with our own until one or the other's 'head' fell off. We also used to make soldier guns by looping the stem of the plantain around itself just under the head, and then, holding the loop tight in the left hand, sharply pull the stem and shoot the head off, just like a bullet.

Many a happy summer afternoon was passed playing these simple games and little did we know that the bruised leaves of the very same plant, if applied to a bleeding wound, will help to stop the bleeding and bring relief. Certainly plantain could be called a soldier's plant for more than one reason.

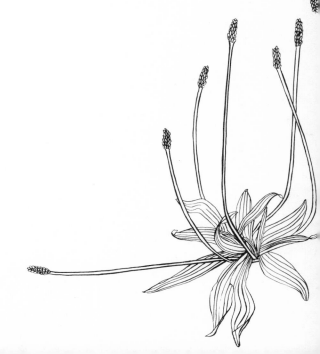

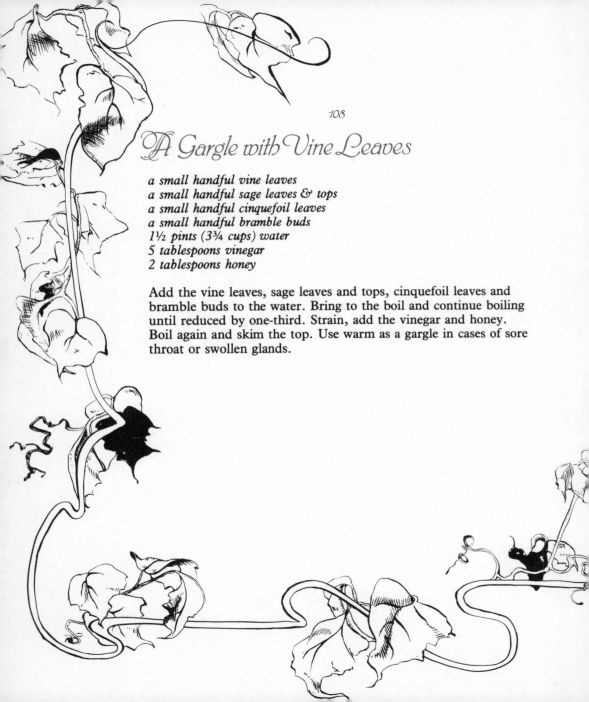

A Gargle with Vine Leaves

a small handful vine leaves
a small handful sage leaves & tops
a small handful cinquefoil leaves
a small handful bramble buds
1½ pints (3¾ cups) water
5 tablespoons vinegar
2 tablespoons honey

Add the vine leaves, sage leaves and tops, cinquefoil leaves and
bramble buds to the water. Bring to the boil and continue boiling
until reduced by one-third. Strain, add the vinegar and honey.
Boil again and skim the top. Use warm as a gargle in cases of sore
throat or swollen glands.

Sage & Honey Gargle

Sage is a powerful healing herb that has been used for over 2000 years to cure all manner of ills from snakebite to the palsy to baldness. Here, it is used as a soothing, antiseptic gargle to ease a sore throat. The cayenne is rich in vitamin C but it must be used very sparingly as it is very hot and pungent.

1 pint (2½ cups) water
1 handful sage leaves & tops
1 tablespoon honey
a pinch of cayenne

Bring the water to the boil and pour over the sage. Leave to stand for 10 minutes. Strain, stir in the honey and cayenne. Use, warm, to gargle as often as desired.

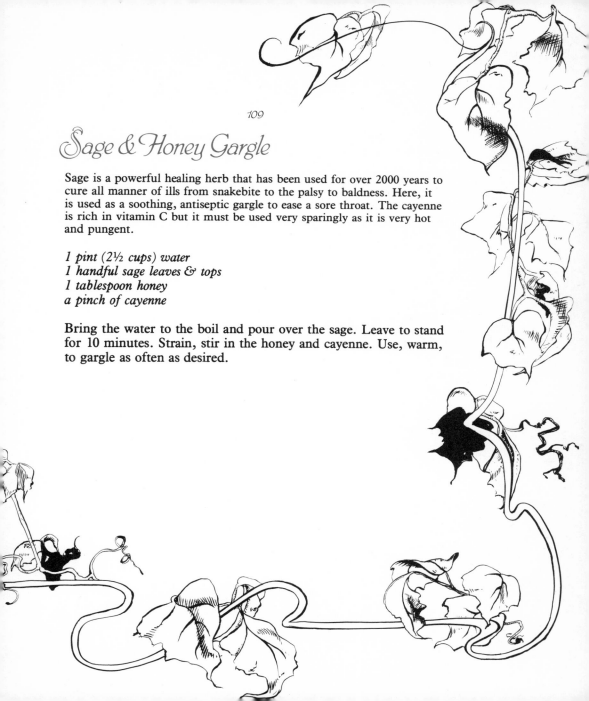

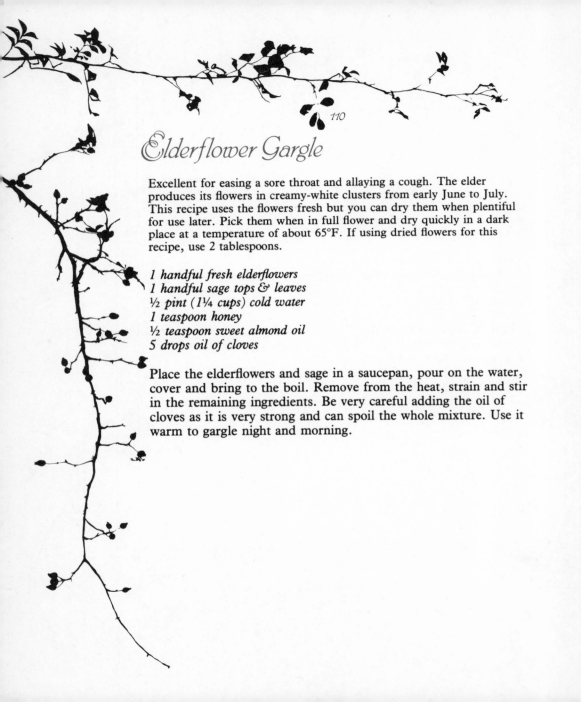

Elderflower Gargle

Excellent for easing a sore throat and allaying a cough. The elder produces its flowers in creamy-white clusters from early June to July. This recipe uses the flowers fresh but you can dry them when plentiful for use later. Pick them when in full flower and dry quickly in a dark place at a temperature of about 65°F. If using dried flowers for this recipe, use 2 tablespoons.

1 handful fresh elderflowers
1 handful sage tops & leaves
½ pint (1¼ cups) cold water
1 teaspoon honey
½ teaspoon sweet almond oil
5 drops oil of cloves

Place the elderflowers and sage in a saucepan, pour on the water, cover and bring to the boil. Remove from the heat, strain and stir in the remaining ingredients. Be very careful adding the oil of cloves as it is very strong and can spoil the whole mixture. Use it warm to gargle night and morning.

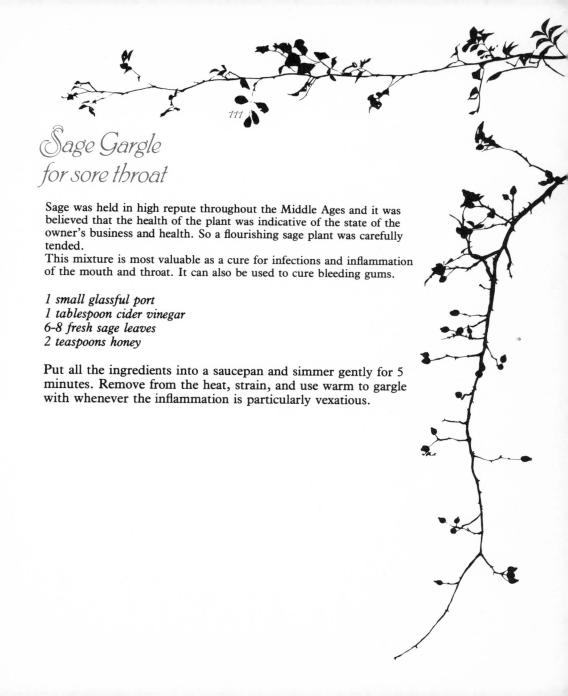

Sage Gargle
for sore throat

Sage was held in high repute throughout the Middle Ages and it was believed that the health of the plant was indicative of the state of the owner's business and health. So a flourishing sage plant was carefully tended.

This mixture is most valuable as a cure for infections and inflammation of the mouth and throat. It can also be used to cure bleeding gums.

1 small glassful port
1 tablespoon cider vinegar
6-8 fresh sage leaves
2 teaspoons honey

Put all the ingredients into a saucepan and simmer gently for 5 minutes. Remove from the heat, strain, and use warm to gargle with whenever the inflammation is particularly vexatious.

Herbal Bath Vinegar

Bath vinegars are both invigorating and antiseptic, so are particularly beneficial for those who are feeling under the weather.

½ pint (1 cup) cider vinegar
½ pint (1 cup) water
3 tablespoons dried herbs, chosen from basil, mint, lemon balm, thyme, marjoram

Bring the vinegar and water to the boil. Add the herbs and remove from the heat. Leave to steep for at least 8 hours, preferably overnight. Strain into a screw-topped jar. Use 1 cupful per bath.

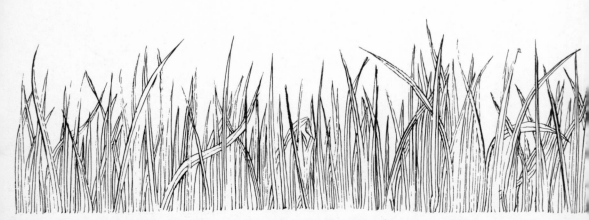

Herb & Oatmeal Bag
for the bath

Oatmeal softens the water and herbs scent it and release their natural oils to soothe and relax. Lavender has been used for thousands of years, not only for its fragrance but also for its disinfectant and soothing qualities. Any of the other aromatic herbs can be used along with the lavender – a friend particularly recommends yarrow.

2 handfuls oatmeal
a small handful fresh or dried lavender flowers and tops
1 handful mixed herbs, preferably thyme, rosemary, lemon balm, yarrow

Combine the ingredients and place in the centre of a square of muslin. Gather up the corners and tie tightly to make a bag. Hold this under the full force of the running taps. Don't have the water too hot as it is more relaxing to bathe in warm water. Use the oatmeal bag to rub all over your body to clean, soften and nourish the skin, but be careful of any sharp twigs among the herbs or else you will end up scratching yourself all over.

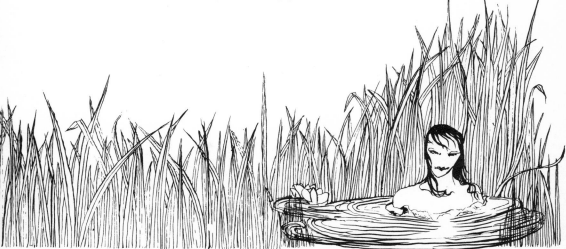

A Sleep-inducing Pillow

Take a warm herbal bath (see page 113) before retiring and have this aromatic bag under your pillow to soothe and relax the nerves and induce sleep. If you use dried herbs the aroma lasts longer and can be revived by adding a few drops of essential oil to the mixture inside.

½ cup dried hops
½ cup dried lavender
½ cup dried lemon thyme or lemon balm

Mix all the ingredients together and fill a small muslin bag. Place under your pillow.
Another good tip is to lie in bed with the head pointing towards the north so that the earth's magnetic currents will inspire soothing rhythms to send you off to sleep.

A Cure for Sprains

1 handful fresh sage leaves
¼ pint (⅔ cup) vinegar

Bruise the sage leaves and add them to the vinegar in a saucepan.
Bring to the boil and simmer for 5 minutes. Remove from the
heat, steep a cloth in the liquid and apply it folded and as hot as
can be borne, to the affected part.

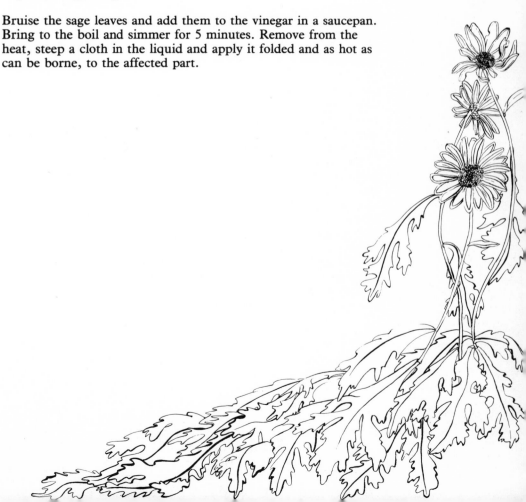

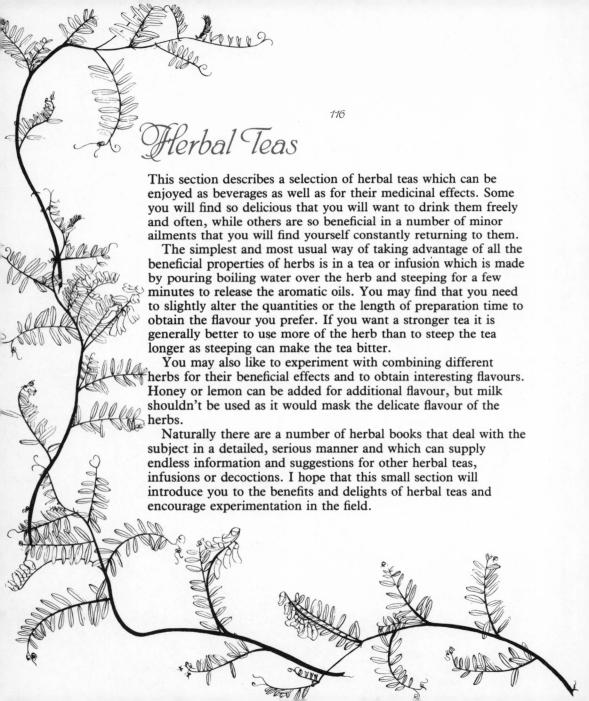

Herbal Teas

This section describes a selection of herbal teas which can be enjoyed as beverages as well as for their medicinal effects. Some you will find so delicious that you will want to drink them freely and often, while others are so beneficial in a number of minor ailments that you will find yourself constantly returning to them.

The simplest and most usual way of taking advantage of all the beneficial properties of herbs is in a tea or infusion which is made by pouring boiling water over the herb and steeping for a few minutes to release the aromatic oils. You may find that you need to slightly alter the quantities or the length of preparation time to obtain the flavour you prefer. If you want a stronger tea it is generally better to use more of the herb than to steep the tea longer as steeping can make the tea bitter.

You may also like to experiment with combining different herbs for their beneficial effects and to obtain interesting flavours. Honey or lemon can be added for additional flavour, but milk shouldn't be used as it would mask the delicate flavour of the herbs.

Naturally there are a number of herbal books that deal with the subject in a detailed, serious manner and which can supply endless information and suggestions for other herbal teas, infusions or decoctions. I hope that this small section will introduce you to the benefits and delights of herbal teas and encourage experimentation in the field.

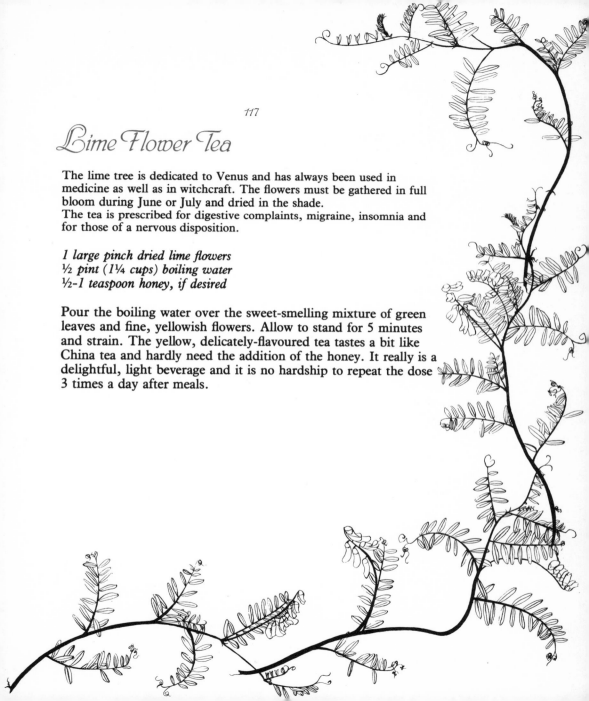

Lime Flower Tea

The lime tree is dedicated to Venus and has always been used in medicine as well as in witchcraft. The flowers must be gathered in full bloom during June or July and dried in the shade.
The tea is prescribed for digestive complaints, migraine, insomnia and for those of a nervous disposition.

1 large pinch dried lime flowers
½ pint (1¼ cups) boiling water
½-1 teaspoon honey, if desired

Pour the boiling water over the sweet-smelling mixture of green leaves and fine, yellowish flowers. Allow to stand for 5 minutes and strain. The yellow, delicately-flavoured tea tastes a bit like China tea and hardly need the addition of the honey. It really is a delightful, light beverage and it is no hardship to repeat the dose 3 times a day after meals.

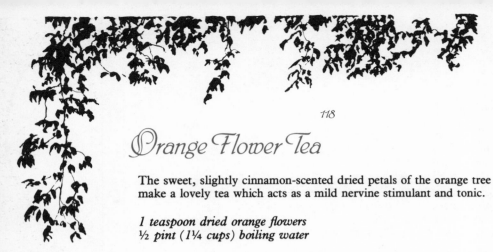

Orange Flower Tea

The sweet, slightly cinnamon-scented dried petals of the orange tree make a lovely tea which acts as a mild nervine stimulant and tonic.

1 teaspoon dried orange flowers
½ pint (1¼ cups) boiling water

Pour the boiling water on to the orange flowers and leave to infuse for 5 minutes. Strain off the pale brown liquid, sweeten with ½ teaspoon honey if desired, and take 1 cupful 2 or 3 times a day.

Birch Tea

This should be made from the young leaves of the birch tree which are full of vitamin C. It is a wonderful tonic for those whose systems are sluggish after the winter. If taken 3 times a day for a month, it should cure a spotty skin or dull complexion.

Take a pinch of the fresh leaves or 1 teaspoon of dried ones, add ½ pint (1¼ cups) boiling water and allow to stand for 8 minutes. Strain and drink the rather pleasant, green, woody-flavoured tea 3 times a day.

Comfrey Tea

The leaves of this marvellous plant, when made into an infusion and taken internally, is a powerful remedy for coughs, sinusitis, asthma and lung disorders.

1 tablespoon dried comfrey leaves
½ pint (1¼ cups) boiling water

Pour the boiling water over the dried leaves and allow to steep for 10 minutes. The resulting greenish brown liquid has a not unpleasant woody taste which is perhaps improved by the addition of ½ teaspoon honey. The tea should be taken 3 times a day.

Infusion of Comfrey Root

This remedy is excellent for enteritis, dysentery and stomach ulcers as the famous attributes of comfrey "favour the development and growth of new tissues" both inside the body as well as externally.

2 ounces (½ cup) fresh comfrey root, chopped
1 pint (2½ cups) water

Pour the water over the chopped root in a basin and leave to infuse in a cool place for 3-4 hours. Strain and take a small cupful 3-4 times a day.

Angelica Tea

The 'angelic' herb is so-called from a belief in its medicinal virtues especially against plague and pestilence – it was chewed during the Great Plague of 1665 to avoid infection. It was also used as a protector against spirits and witches.

The infusion which eases flatulence and soothes the digestion, can be made either from the root of the plant which yields a pale brown, acrid tea or else from the leaves which gives a pale green, much more pleasant-tasting tea. The candied stem used in confectionery should not be used.

Take 1 teaspoon of the dried leaves or root, pour on ½ pint (1¼ cups) boiling water and leave for 5 minutes. Strain. You will probably need to add honey if you use the root. Take 1 cupful of the tea, 3 times a day.

Witch Hazel Tea

A tea made from witch hazel is unsurpassed in treating internal bleeding from the lungs, stomach, uterus or bowels. It arrests excessive menstruation and is good in cases of diarrhoea. For a nose bleed the tea should be sniffed up the nose.

1 large pinch dried witch hazel leaves
½ pint (1¼ cups) boiling water
1 teaspoon honey

Pour the boiling water over the dried leaves and leave to infuse for 8-10 minutes. Strain off the yellow-green liquid with its rather boring, woody taste, add the honey to liven it up and take a cupful 4 times a day.

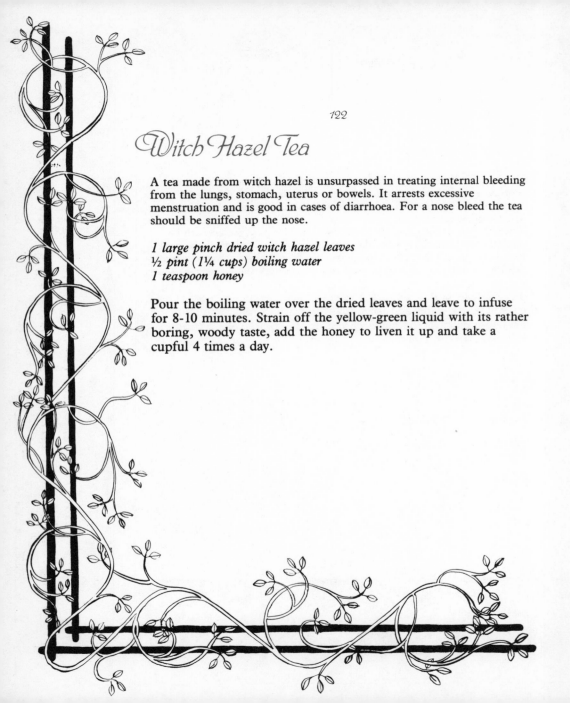

Borage Tea

In the 16th century, borage had a great reputation as a cheering herb and according to Gerard it gives courage. When taken as a tea it acts quickly to lift a slight depression and can also be used to reduce a fever. I find the tea made with dried borage leaves smells strongly of seaweed and is not very pleasant. The addition of a teaspoon of honey and a slice of lemon does improve the flavour, but I'm still not very fond of it.

The proportions are 1 teaspoon of the dried leaves to ½ pint (1¼ cups) boiling water, infused for 5 minutes and taken 4 or 5 times a day.

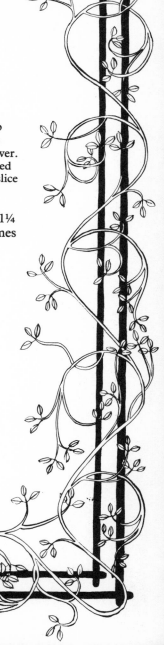

Camomile Tea

This is a favourite herbal tea, particularly in Switzerland and Germany, although personally I find the smell and flavour rather unpleasant and too strong to make it a palatable drink. Perhaps it is an acquired taste. The tea is beneficial for a sluggish digestion, flatulence, digestive disorders and insomnia.

Pour ½ pint (1¼ cups) boiling water over 1 teaspoon of the dried flowers. Leave for 5 minutes before straining. The addition of 1 teaspoon each of lemon juice and honey does improve the flavour but doesn't do much for the smell.

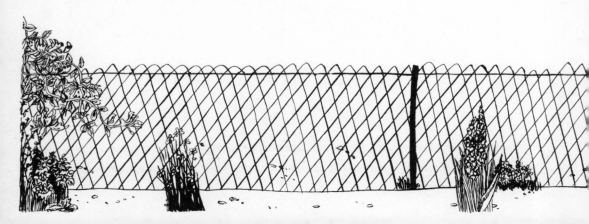

Nettle Tea

The nettle is anti-asthmatic – the juice of the leaves or root when mixed with honey will bring welcome relief to bronchitis or asthma sufferers. The dried leaves burnt and the smoke inhaled through the mouth will have the same effect.

Nettles should be gathered on a fine day in spring, just before they come into bloom, and then dried in a cool, airy place.

This tea is a fine general tonic that also stimulates the digestive functions.

2 teaspoons dried nettle leaves
½ pint (1¼ cups) boiling water

Pour the boiling water over the dried leaves and allow to infuse for 6-8 minutes. Strain off the pale green tea with its woody taste and take as often as you like. You can add a slice of lemon and a teaspoon of honey if you wish.

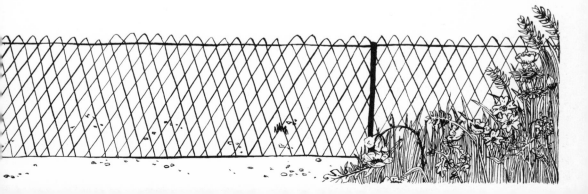

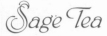

Sage Tea

In its natural state sage is very like garden sage, only shrubbier, and it grows wild all along the Mediterranean coast. An important cottage industry in Dalmatia is the growing of sage, not only for its sale as a herb but also for its flowers which attract the bees who then produce the most wonderful sage honey – a speciality that commands the highest price.

This tea is a pleasant drink and an admirable cleanser and purifier of the blood. It is also good for weakness of the stomach and digestion.

2 pints (5 cups) boiling water
½ ounce (½ cup) fresh sage leaves
1 ounce (2 tablespoons) sugar
juice of 1 lemon

Pour the boiling water over the other ingredients, stir well and leave to stand in a warm place for 30 minutes. Strain and take warm, in small frequent doses.

Lemon Balm Tea

Culpeper said of lemon balm that "it causeth the mind and heart to become merry . . . and driveth away all troublesome cares and thoughts." This tea is excellent for nausea and vomiting and will quieten and settle the stomach. It is particularly recommended for painful menstruation as it eases the cramps.

1 teaspoon dried lemon balm
½ pint (1¼ cups) boiling water
1 teaspoon honey
1 slice lemon

Pour the water over the sweet, lemon-scented leaves. Let stand for 5 minutes before straining off the greenish-brown liquid. Stir in the honey and add the slice of lemon. Take 4 cupfuls a day, or 6 a day if treating menstrual cramps.

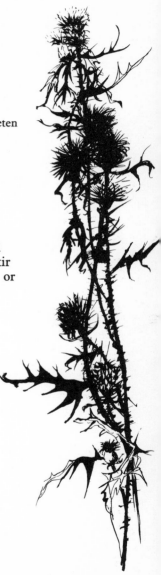

Elecampane Tea

Elecampane was formerly used to confer immortality and to cure
wounds. In addition to these virtues, a tea made from its hard, horny
root which is the only part of the plant that is used, also cures coughs
and colds. It also has a beneficial effect on digestive and menstrual
disorders.

1 teaspoon elecampane
½ pint (1¼ cups) boiling water
1 teaspoon honey

Pour the boiling water over the brown chips of elecampane root.
Leave for 5 minutes then strain off the yellowish-brown liquid
which has a rather sharp taste. Sweeten with honey and take 1
cupful 3 times a day before meals.

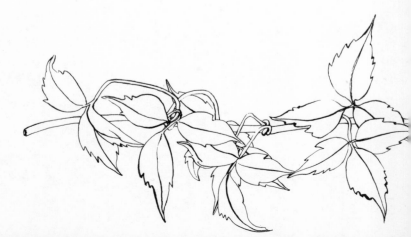

Parsley Tea

Parsley is rich in iron and vitamins. This infusion aids digestion and relieves the cramps that often accompany menstruation.

¾ pint (2 cups) water
1 large handful fresh parsley, leaves and stalks

Bring the water to the boil, pour over the parsley and leave to infuse for about 10 minutes. Strain. Take a small cupful 3 or 4 times a day. The tea can be slightly sweetened with honey if desired.

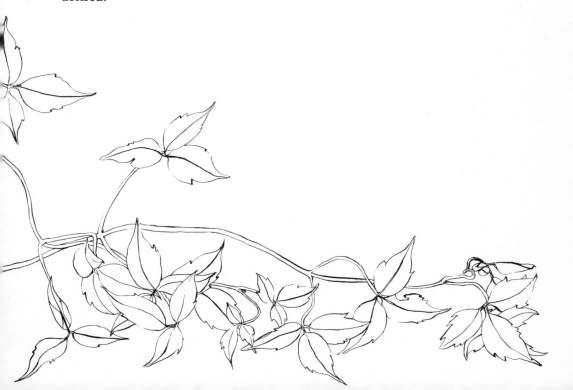

Infusion of Basil
to allay nausea

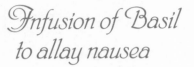

The Ancient Greeks and Romans both firmly believed that it was essential to hurl abuse at a plant of basil to ensure its strong and healthy growth.

The herbalists of old couldn't agree as to its medicinal value, but it was said to inspire love and sympathy between human beings.

This infusion can be used for mild nervous disorders and has been used to effect in cases of morning sickness during pregnancy, arresting vomiting and allaying the feelings of nausea.

1 pint (2½ cups) boiling water
1 handful fresh basil, stalks & leaves

Pour the boiling water over the herb and allow to infuse for 15 minutes. Strain, and take freely during the day, especially when nausea is most often felt (ie in the mornings).

Blackberry Antidote to dysentery

The bark of the root and the leaves of the blackberry have long been esteemed as excellent astringents and tonic, proving a valuable remedy for dysentery and diarrhoea. The fruit too, can be taken freely and at one time these berries alone were considered a fine cure for dysentery.

To make a decoction it is better to use the dried leaves which are more aromatic than fresh ones. Use 1 ounce (½ cup) of the dried leaves to 1 pint (2½ cups) boiling water and steep for 15 minutes before straining and using. The does is 1 tablespoon 4 or 5 times a day.

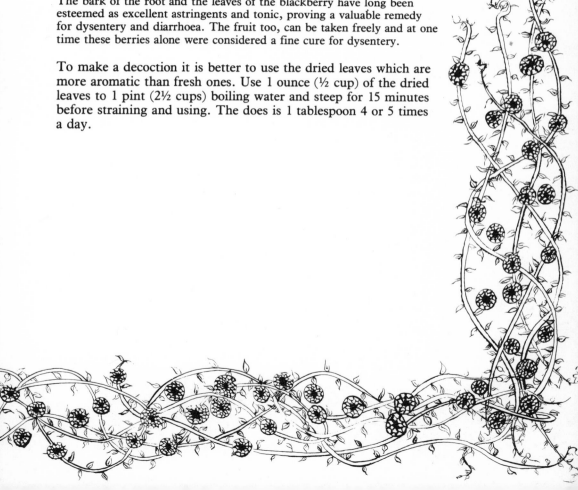

To Cure Diarrhoea
in children

An infusion of raspberry leaves, taken cold, is a reliable remedy for diarrhoea and stomach disorders in adults as well as children, but it is mild enough even for babies under one year old when given in small doses.

1 ounce (½ cup) dried raspberry leaves
1 pint (2½ cups) boiling water
1-inch piece of stick cinnamon

Put the raspberry leaves into a saucepan, add the boiling water and stick cinnamon and simmer for about 30 minutes. Strain and cool. The dose for a child under 1 year is ½ teaspoon 4 times a day; for a child over 1 year give 1 teaspoon.

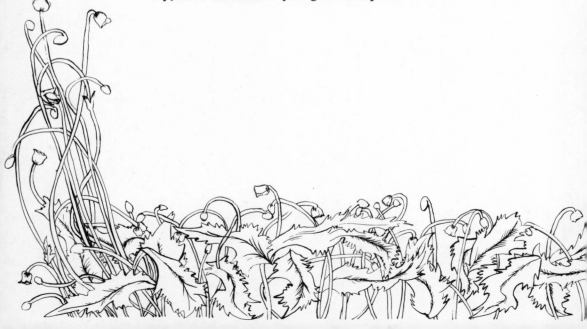

Raspberry Leaf Tea
to assist in childbirth

For countless years raspberry leaf tea has been prescribed during the last weeks of pregnancy to ensure an easy and quick labour, and a speedy recovery. For robust mothers the tea should be taken regularly for the final 5 or 6 weeks, and those of a more delicate disposition should start the treatment 3 months before the expected birth.

1 teaspoon dried raspberry leaves
½ pint (1¼ cups) boiling water

Infuse the dried leaves in the boiling water for 20 minutes. Strain, sweeten if required with honey, and take freely, warm, at least 3 times a day.

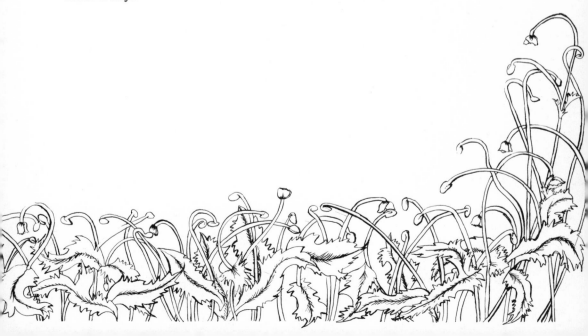

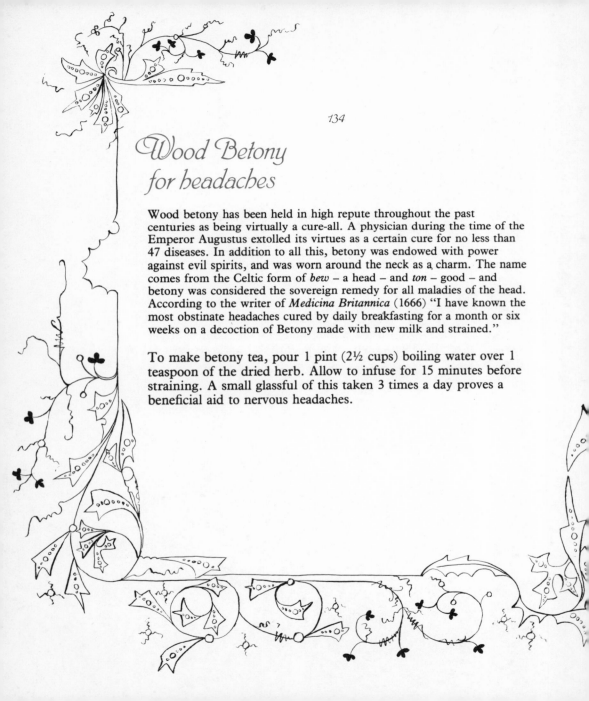

Wood Betony
for headaches

Wood betony has been held in high repute throughout the past
centuries as being virtually a cure-all. A physician during the time of the
Emperor Augustus extolled its virtues as a certain cure for no less than
47 diseases. In addition to all this, betony was endowed with power
against evil spirits, and was worn around the neck as a charm. The name
comes from the Celtic form of *bew* – a head – and *ton* – good – and
betony was considered the sovereign remedy for all maladies of the head.
According to the writer of *Medicina Britannica* (1666) "I have known the
most obstinate headaches cured by daily breakfasting for a month or six
weeks on a decoction of Betony made with new milk and strained."

To make betony tea, pour 1 pint (2½ cups) boiling water over 1
teaspoon of the dried herb. Allow to infuse for 15 minutes before
straining. A small glassful of this taken 3 times a day proves a
beneficial aid to nervous headaches.

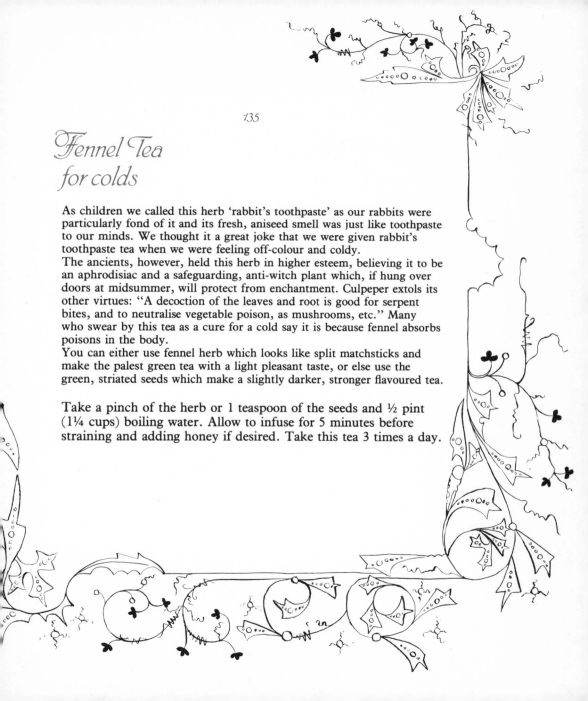

Fennel Tea
for colds

As children we called this herb 'rabbit's toothpaste' as our rabbits were particularly fond of it and its fresh, aniseed smell was just like toothpaste to our minds. We thought it a great joke that we were given rabbit's toothpaste tea when we were feeling off-colour and coldy.

The ancients, however, held this herb in higher esteem, believing it to be an aphrodisiac and a safeguarding, anti-witch plant which, if hung over doors at midsummer, will protect from enchantment. Culpeper extols its other virtues: "A decoction of the leaves and root is good for serpent bites, and to neutralise vegetable poison, as mushrooms, etc." Many who swear by this tea as a cure for a cold say it is because fennel absorbs poisons in the body.

You can either use fennel herb which looks like split matchsticks and make the palest green tea with a light pleasant taste, or else use the green, striated seeds which make a slightly darker, stronger flavoured tea.

Take a pinch of the herb or 1 teaspoon of the seeds and ½ pint (1¼ cups) boiling water. Allow to infuse for 5 minutes before straining and adding honey if desired. Take this tea 3 times a day.

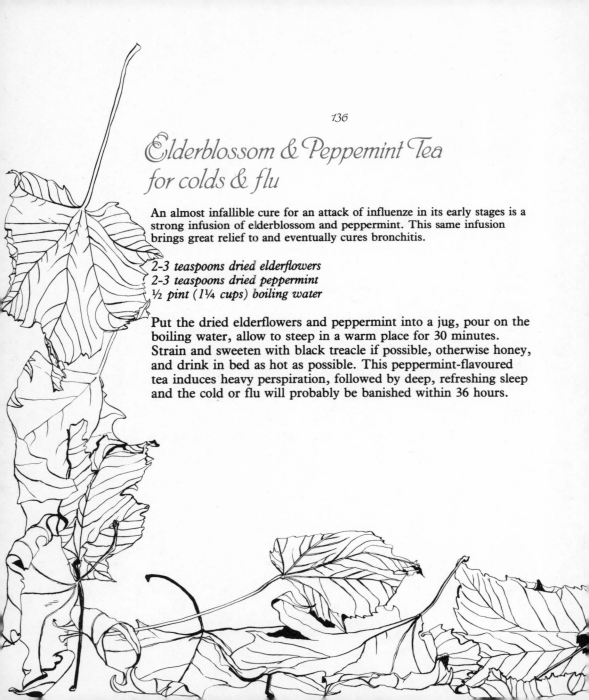

Elderblossom & Peppemint Tea
for colds & flu

An almost infallible cure for an attack of influenze in its early stages is a strong infusion of elderblossom and peppermint. This same infusion brings great relief to and eventually cures bronchitis.

2-3 teaspoons dried elderflowers
2-3 teaspoons dried peppermint
½ pint (1¼ cups) boiling water

Put the dried elderflowers and peppermint into a jug, pour on the boiling water, allow to steep in a warm place for 30 minutes. Strain and sweeten with black treacle if possible, otherwise honey, and drink in bed as hot as possible. This peppermint-flavoured tea induces heavy perspiration, followed by deep, refreshing sleep and the cold or flu will probably be banished within 36 hours.

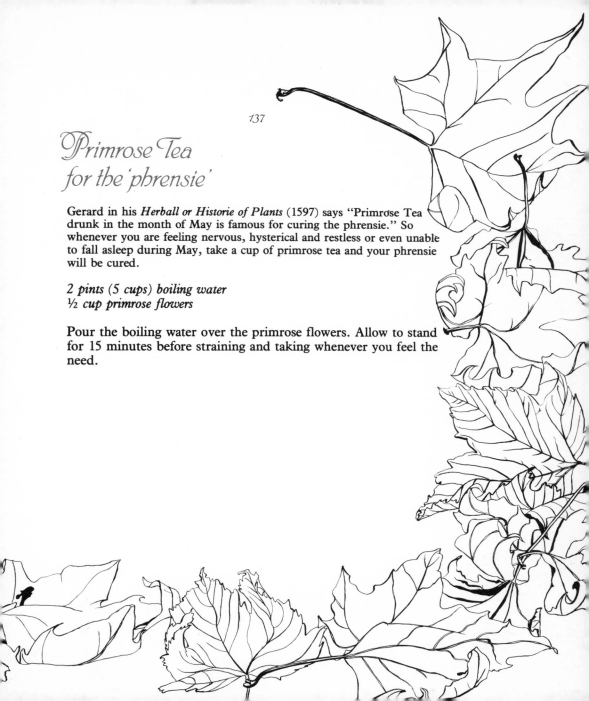

Primrose Tea
for the 'phrensie'

Gerard in his *Herball or Historie of Plants* (1597) says "Primrose Tea drunk in the month of May is famous for curing the phrensie." So whenever you are feeling nervous, hysterical and restless or even unable to fall asleep during May, take a cup of primrose tea and your phrensie will be cured.

2 pints (5 cups) boiling water
½ cup primrose flowers

Pour the boiling water over the primrose flowers. Allow to stand for 15 minutes before straining and taking whenever you feel the need.

Yarrow Tea

The bruised leaves of yarrow were formerly considered an excellent remedy to stop wounds bleeding. Gerard tells us that it got its name *Achillea* because Achilles used the plant to staunch the bleeding wounds of his soldiers. In the Highlands of Scotland they still make an ointment from it which they apply to wounds.

Yarrow tea is a good remedy for severe colds as it opens the pores and purifies the blood and is particularly recommended in the early stages of children's colds and in measles and other eruptive diseases.

1 pint (2½ cups) boiling water
1 tablespoon dried yarrow
1 tablespoon honey

Pour the boiling water over the herb, allow to stand for 10 minutes before straining and sweetening with honey. The tea should be taken warm in small glassfuls 3 or 4 times daily.

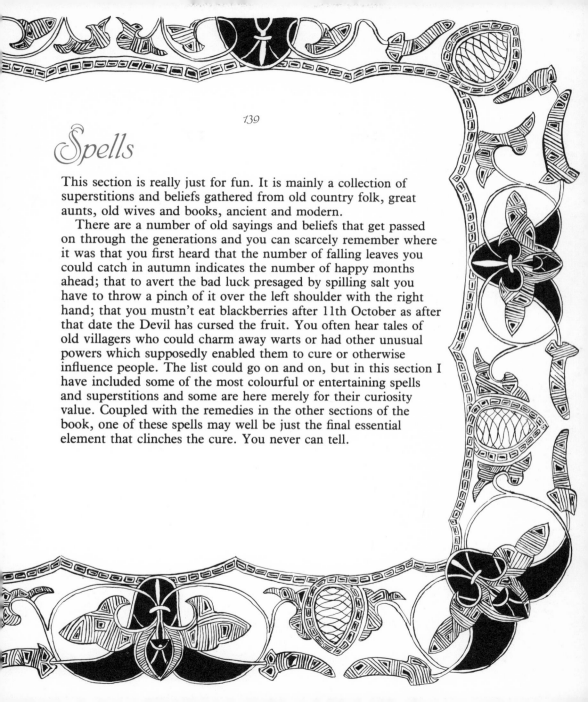

Spells

This section is really just for fun. It is mainly a collection of
superstitions and beliefs gathered from old country folk, great
aunts, old wives and books, ancient and modern.

There are a number of old sayings and beliefs that get passed
on through the generations and you can scarcely remember where
it was that you first heard that the number of falling leaves you
could catch in autumn indicates the number of happy months
ahead; that to avert the bad luck presaged by spilling salt you
have to throw a pinch of it over the left shoulder with the right
hand; that you mustn't eat blackberries after 11th October as after
that date the Devil has cursed the fruit. You often hear tales of
old villagers who could charm away warts or had other unusual
powers which supposedly enabled them to cure or otherwise
influence people. The list could go on and on, but in this section I
have included some of the most colourful or entertaining spells
and superstitions and some are here merely for their curiosity
value. Coupled with the remedies in the other sections of the
book, one of these spells may well be just the final essential
element that clinches the cure. You never can tell.

Spell
to bring good fortune

If you were born under a full moon and fall upon hard times, you can call upon Diana to help you. Gaze at the moon while repeating these words and the number of coins in your pocket should magically double.

"Moon, Moon, beautiful Moon!
Fairer far than any star;
Moon, O Moon, if it may be,
Bring good fortune unto me!"

To Ward Off Evil Spirits

Mistletoe was worshipped by the Druids who were the only ones in ancient times who were allowed to gather it. They went forth dressed in white robes to search for the sacred plant, and when it was discovered, one of the Druids climbed the tree and cut the mistletoe away from its host tree with a golden knife.

To hang a twig of the mistletoe around the neck wards off evil spirits but it is essential that no part of the plant ever touches the ground as some of its efficacy will thereby be lost.

To Avoid Intoxication

Ivy was held in high esteem by the ancients and it was dedicated to Bacchus, the god of wine, who is often represented as a fine, bearded man with black eyes and flowing locks crowned with a wreath of ivy. Hence the growth of the belief that the way to avoid intoxication was to bind the brow with ivy.

Old writers also tell us that one can avoid the effects of drinking too much by steeping a handful of bruised ivy leaves in a jug of wine prior to drinking it.

Love Potion

Coriander seeds are spicy, sweet and orangey and impart a delicious flavour to the wine in this love potion. The Chinese believed these seeds to have the power of conferring immortality on those who partook of them, which no doubt strengthens the power of the potion.

A pinch of the ground seeds must be stirred into a glass of good, mature red wine while this chant is repeated

"Warm seed, warm heart
Let us never be apart."

and as the wine is drunk a warm and enduring passion will be aroused.

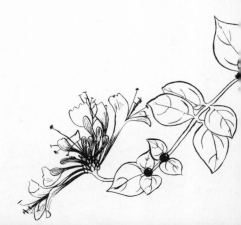

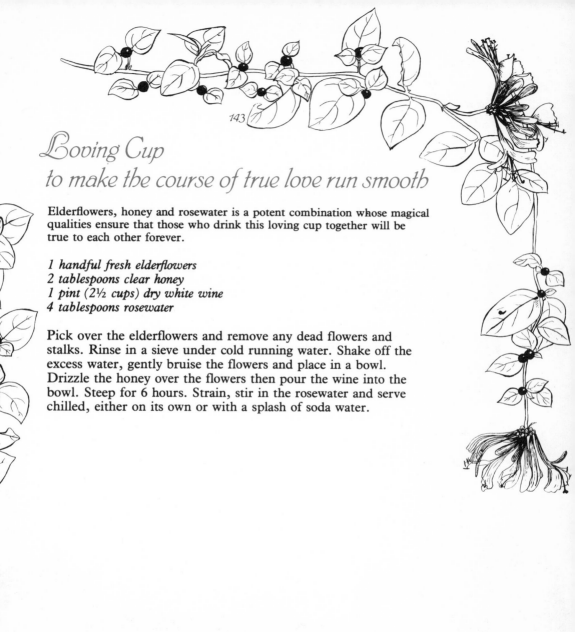

Loving Cup
to make the course of true love run smooth

Elderflowers, honey and rosewater is a potent combination whose magical qualities ensure that those who drink this loving cup together will be true to each other forever.

1 handful fresh elderflowers
2 tablespoons clear honey
1 pint (2½ cups) dry white wine
4 tablespoons rosewater

Pick over the elderflowers and remove any dead flowers and stalks. Rinse in a sieve under cold running water. Shake off the excess water, gently bruise the flowers and place in a bowl. Drizzle the honey over the flowers then pour the wine into the bowl. Steep for 6 hours. Strain, stir in the rosewater and serve chilled, either on its own or with a splash of soda water.

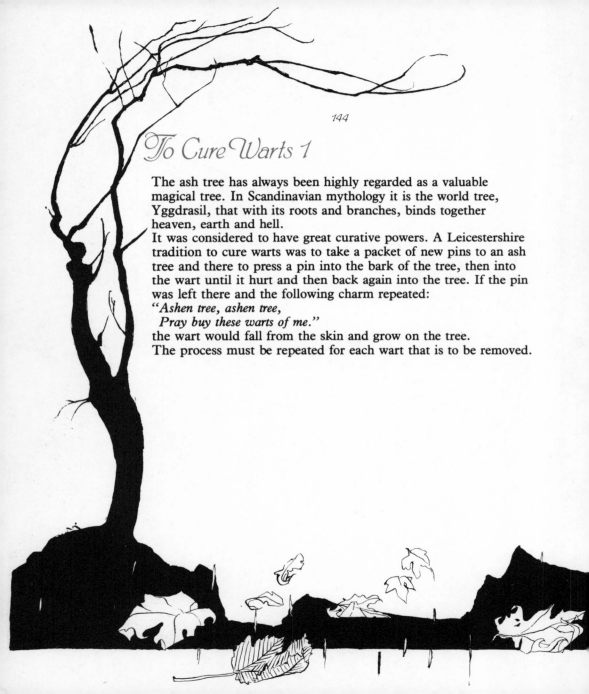

To Cure Warts 1

The ash tree has always been highly regarded as a valuable
magical tree. In Scandinavian mythology it is the world tree,
Yggdrasil, that with its roots and branches, binds together
heaven, earth and hell.

It was considered to have great curative powers. A Leicestershire
tradition to cure warts was to take a packet of new pins to an ash
tree and there to press a pin into the bark of the tree, then into
the wart until it hurt and then back again into the tree. If the pin
was left there and the following charm repeated:

"Ashen tree, ashen tree,
  Pray buy these warts of me."

the wart would fall from the skin and grow on the tree.

The process must be repeated for each wart that is to be removed.

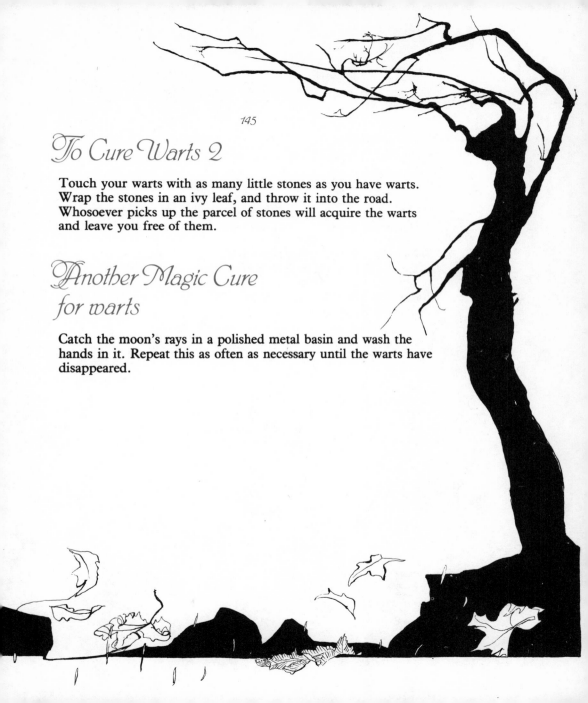

To Cure Warts 2

Touch your warts with as many little stones as you have warts. Wrap the stones in an ivy leaf, and throw it into the road. Whosoever picks up the parcel of stones will acquire the warts and leave you free of them.

Another Magic Cure for warts

Catch the moon's rays in a polished metal basin and wash the hands in it. Repeat this as often as necessary until the warts have disappeared.

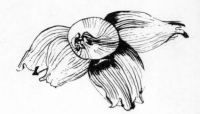

To Cure Toothache

Marcellus swore by this cure.

Stand booted on the ground under the open sky. Catch a frog by the head; spit into its mouth and ask it to take away the ache.

If a needle is run through a wood-louse and immediately the aching tooth touched with that needle, it will cease to ache.

Repeat the following spell which was found to be very efficacious: *"Galbes, Galbat, Galdes, Galdat."*

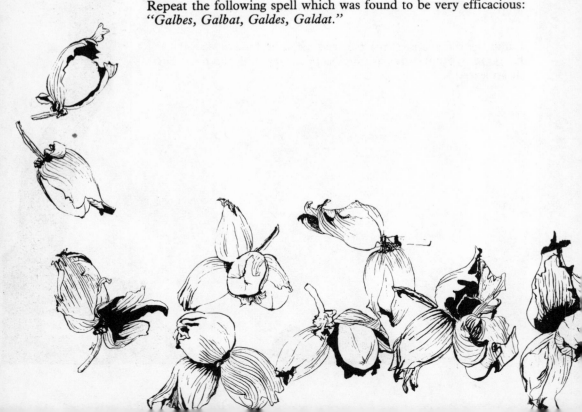

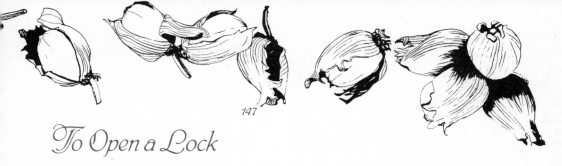

To Open a Lock

If a door lock is jammed a sure way of gaining access is to force a sprig of wild chicory into the lock before attempting to turn the key.

Headache Cure

Pliny advocated this remedy: Gather a plant that is growing on the head of a statue, being careful not to let it touch the ground. Attach it to a red string or tape and wear it round the neck.

A Lucky Sneeze

Aristotle said that to sneeze from noon to midnight was fortunate, but from midnight to noon was unlucky.

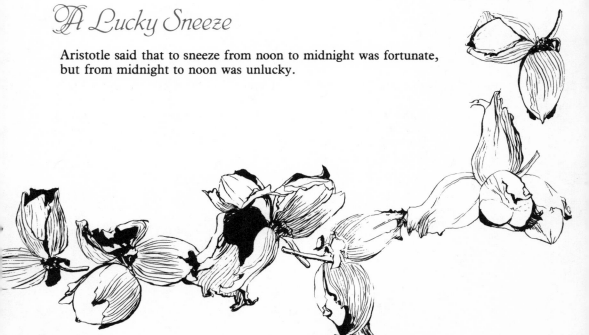

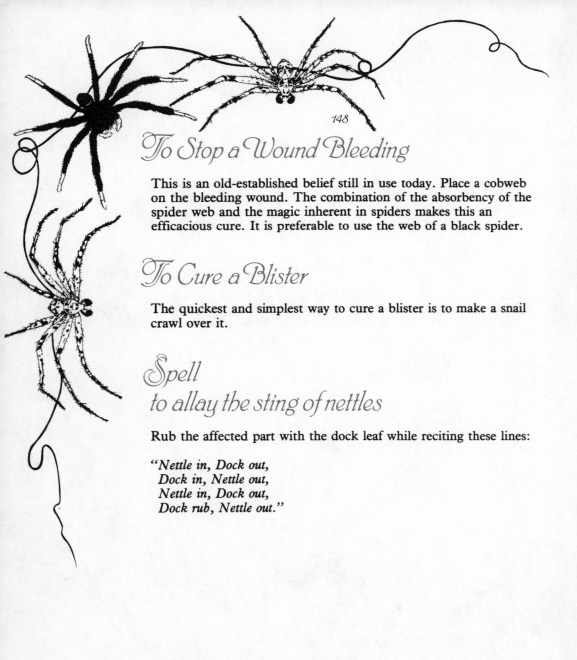

To Stop a Wound Bleeding

This is an old-established belief still in use today. Place a cobweb on the bleeding wound. The combination of the absorbency of the spider web and the magic inherent in spiders makes this an efficacious cure. It is preferable to use the web of a black spider.

To Cure a Blister

The quickest and simplest way to cure a blister is to make a snail crawl over it.

Spell
to allay the sting of nettles

Rub the affected part with the dock leaf while reciting these lines:

"Nettle in, Dock out,
  Dock in, Nettle out,
  Nettle in, Dock out,
  Dock rub, Nettle out."

Sussex Cure
for ague

Place the leaves of the tansy into the shoes for a sure cure of the ague.

Ashmole's Cure
for ague

Ashmole the astrologer wrote in 1661:
"I took early in the morning a good dose of elixir and hung three spiders about my neck; they drove my ague away."

When you next have a fever it might be worth trying Ashmole's cure as a last resort before reaching for the aspirins.

To Stave Off Rheumatism

At all times carry a potato in the pocket and this will most successfully keep rheumatism at bay.

Ladies in former times had special pockets sewn into their dresses in which to carry a small raw potato just for this purpose.

To Heal à Stye

A stye is a small inflamed swelling on the rim of the eyelid. Some people, especially adolescents, are plagued with these.

An infallible cure is to rub the stye 3 times with a gold wedding ring, or failing that, use the tail of a black cat.

Charm against Magic

Coral was greatly prized as a charm against magic and coral beads were often hung around babies' necks for protection from the Evil Eye.

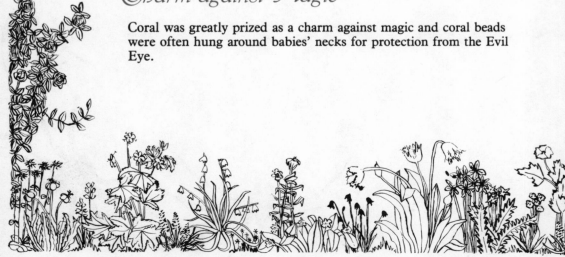

A Certain Cure
for a whitlow

The earth has always been a powerful spell-binder, playing a major part in mortal events, especially those of birth and death. All earth had magical properties but that with the greatest was holy ground such as a churchyard, or a place where three lands meet.

To cure a whitlow, you just stick the sore finger into the ground, the more magical the ground the better. The treatment can be repeated as necessary until the cure is complete.

An Ancient Cure
for pimples

Watch for a shooting star and then as the star is falling in the sky, wipe the pimples with a cloth and throw it to the ground. As the star falls from the sky so the pimples will fall from your body. One precaution is that you must be careful not to wipe the face with your bare hands or the pimples will be transferred to them.

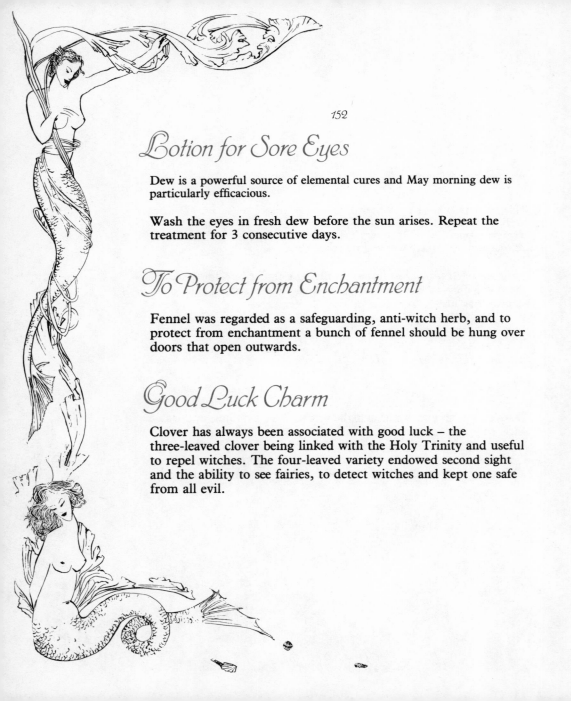

Lotion for Sore Eyes

Dew is a powerful source of elemental cures and May morning dew is particularly efficacious.

Wash the eyes in fresh dew before the sun arises. Repeat the treatment for 3 consecutive days.

To Protect from Enchantment

Fennel was regarded as a safeguarding, anti-witch herb, and to protect from enchantment a bunch of fennel should be hung over doors that open outwards.

Good Luck Charm

Clover has always been associated with good luck – the three-leaved clover being linked with the Holy Trinity and useful to repel witches. The four-leaved variety endowed second sight and the ability to see fairies, to detect witches and kept one safe from all evil.

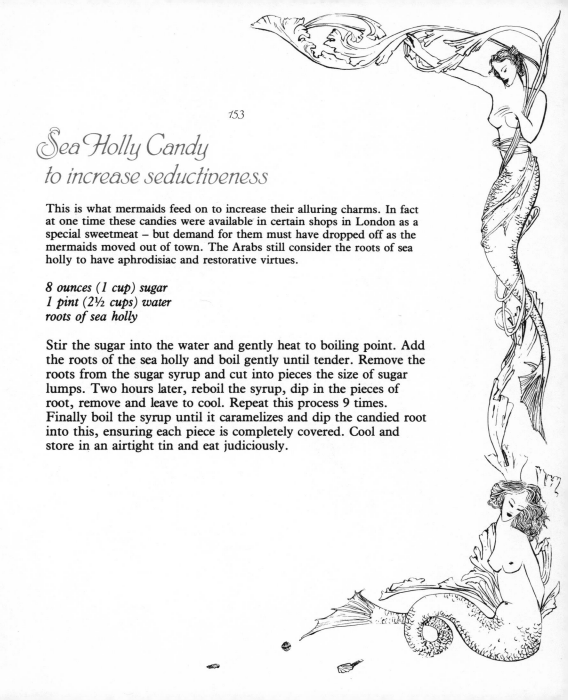

Sea Holly Candy
to increase seductiveness

This is what mermaids feed on to increase their alluring charms. In fact at one time these candies were available in certain shops in London as a special sweetmeat – but demand for them must have dropped off as the mermaids moved out of town. The Arabs still consider the roots of sea holly to have aphrodisiac and restorative virtues.

8 ounces (1 cup) sugar
1 pint (2½ cups) water
roots of sea holly

Stir the sugar into the water and gently heat to boiling point. Add the roots of the sea holly and boil gently until tender. Remove the roots from the sugar syrup and cut into pieces the size of sugar lumps. Two hours later, reboil the syrup, dip in the pieces of root, remove and leave to cool. Repeat this process 9 times. Finally boil the syrup until it caramelizes and dip the candied root into this, ensuring each piece is completely covered. Cool and store in an airtight tin and eat judiciously.

List of Suppliers

Baldwins Herbs
173 Walworth Road
London SE17

Culpeper Ltd
Hadstock Road
Linton
Cambridge CB1 6NJ
(mail order customers only)

Robert Jackson Ltd
170 Piccadilly
London W1

Chalk Farm Nutrition Centre
Chalk Farm Road
London NW1

Borchelt Herb Gardens
474 Carriage Shop Road
East Falmouth, Mass 02536

Meadowbrook Herb Garden
Route 138
Wyoming, RI 02898

Rocky Hollow Herb Farm
Box 354
Sussex, NJ 07461

The Tool Shed Herb Farm
Salem Center
Purdy's Station
NY 10578

Yankee Peddler Herb Farm
Rte 4, Box 76
Highway 36N
Brenham, Texas 77833

Index